Chef

Zipora™

ENTERPRISE

HOW TO USE APP

1. DOWNLOAD FREE APP

TEXT KEYWORD
ZIPORA
TO
25827

App Store | Google play

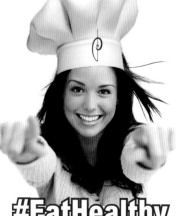

#EatHealthy
with Chef Zipora

2. HOLD APP OVER PHOTOS WITH

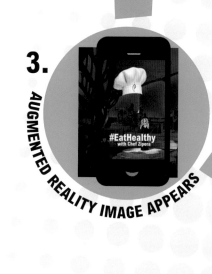

3. AUGMENTED REALITY IMAGE APPEARS

TAKE A SELFIE
& SHARE YOUR HEALTHY

4.

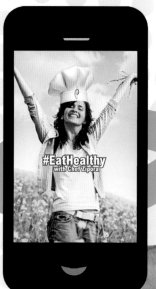

5. POST FUN PHOTOS TO YOUR SOCIALS

TAP IMAGE

6.

UNLOCK SPECIAL INTERACTIVE
CONTENT, OFFERS & VIDEOS
USING THE
INTERACTIVE APP

SPECIAL WEB CONTENT

UNLOCK SPECIAL VIDEOS

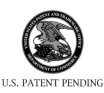

U.S. PATENT PENDING

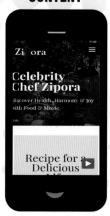

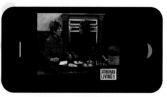

POWERED BY:

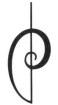

EXPERIENCE CHEF ZIPORA

THIS BOOK CONTAINS INTERACTIVE CONTENT

A Note to the Reader:

I'm all about helping you have incredible experiences. I want you to experience food, flavor, music, health, passion, LIFE in ways beyond what you have before.

One thing we have done to make reading this book more experiential is to embed on several pages some augmented reality images that you can enjoy from your smart phone. These interactive images are noted throughout the book with this symbol ℘. To unlock these special enhanced features, follow the instructions on the adjacent page. ENJOY!

EASY AND FUN TO USE

DOWNLOAD APP   **SCAN PAGE**   **VIDEOS & MORE**

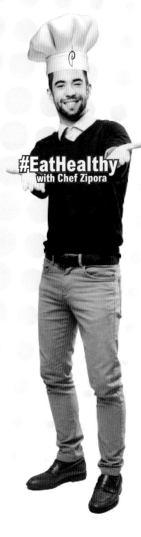

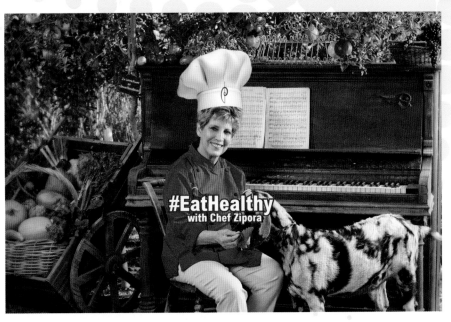

Recipe for a Delicious Life: Discover the Perfect Blend of Food & Music to Stimulate
Your Appetite for Lasting Health, Harmony & Joy!
By Zipora Einav

ISBN-13: 978-0-9994156-1-0 9
ISBN-10: 0999415611 eBook

HigherLife Development Services, Inc.
PO Box 623307
Oviedo, Florida 32762
(407) 563-4806
www.ahigherlife.com

This book is sold with the understanding that the subject matter herein does not constitute professional advice for any specific individual or situation. Opinions in this book are the author's own and don't necessarily represent the publisher.

Chef Zipora, LLC, Inc., Zipora Einav, or HigherLife Development Services, Inc., do not endorse individual vendors, products, or services. Therefore, any reference herein to any vendor, product, or service by trade name, trademark, or manufacturer or otherwise does not constitute or imply the endorsement, recommendation, or approval of this book (Recipe for a Delicious Life), its owners, subsidiaries, partners, or such, in its own.

Printed in the United States of America
10 9 8 7 6 5 4 3 2 1
First Edition

Library of Congress Cataloging-in-Publication Data
Data Control Number: 1-5984789811

Recipe for a
Delicious Life

Discover the Perfect Blend of Food & Music to Stimulate Your Appetite for Lasting Health, Harmony & Joy!

ZIPORA EINAV

MRS. BOB HOPE

August 21, 1997

To whom it may concern,

Please allow this letter to serve as an introduction of Zipora Einav.

Although I have not know Zipora for an extended period of time, I would like to comment on the circumstances of our association. Ms. Einav has assisted with the duties of Personal Chef at the Hope's North Hollywood, California residence for the past three weeks during the absence of our full-time Chef. Our agreement was that this was only a temporary assignment, and upon the return of our permanent employee, the position would cease to exist.

During that brief period, however, Ms. Einav demonstrated her extraordinary ability in the kitchen. Although we did not fully employ her talents as an authority in Spa Cuisine, we nonetheless were treated to samplings of her potential in the realm of health conscience cooking.

Zipora was a great help and performed her duties admirably.

I shall be delighted to answer personally inquiries about her association with the reside

Sincerely,

J. Dennis Paulin
Estate Manager

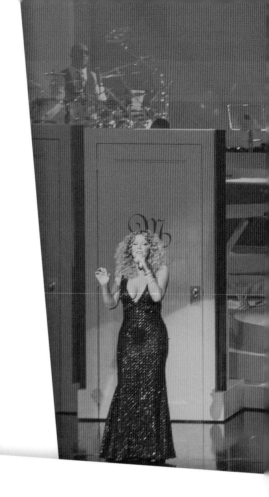

❦ MAROON ENTERTA

To Whom It May Concern:

Please be advised that Zipora Einav was a chef on Mariah Carey's Ra
and an extremely diligent worker. She was a pleasure to work with a
perspective client.

I hope that this information is helpful to you.

Best wishes,

Michael Richardson

Michael Richardson

To Whom It May Concern

Mrs Zipora Einav was working for the Kelly Family for one year.

She prepared lunches and dinners for the whole family and also did the shopping on her own.

She accompanied the Kelly Family on their tours through Germany and Europe and cooked very healthy and palatable food. She took into consideration the wishes of each member of the Kelly Family and also prepared individual meals.

During her time with us Mrs Einav has carried out all duties allocated to her and has been honest and trustworth in her dealings.

She was a good member of our team.

We can highly recommend Mrs Zipora Einav.

KEL-Life Music Production GmbH

Gerd Sparla

Deutsche Bank AG 1 159 565 (BLZ 370 700 60) · Postbank Köln 2 1(
KEL-Life Music Production GmbH. HRB 27 393 AG !

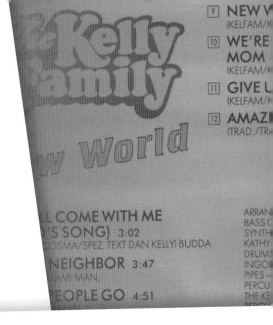

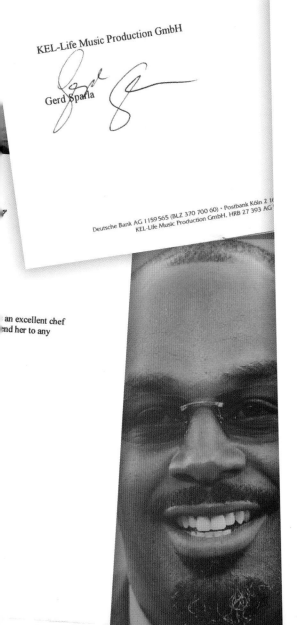

an excellent chef
nd her to any

From the Desk of Mr. & Mrs. Donovan McNabb

August 4, 2010

To Whom It May Concern:

My family has had the pleasure of having celebrity chef Zipora Einav serve as our personal chef from February 2010 through August 2010. Chef Zipora's outstanding meals and her adherence to the Metabolic Typing Diet (MTD) contributed to my husband and I reaching our weight loss goals. With the assistance of Chef Zipora, and the MTD, my husband reported to training camp at his target weight. The diet provided a guideline of appropriate foods that not only encourage weight loss, but also increased our energy levels.

Chef Zipora also took it upon herself to encourage healthy eating habits in our children. As a family, we were very impressed by Chef Zipora's tasty meals and highly recommend her as a personal chef. Chef Zipora's talents and professionalism are second to none.

Sincerely,

Mr. & Mrs. Donovan McNabb

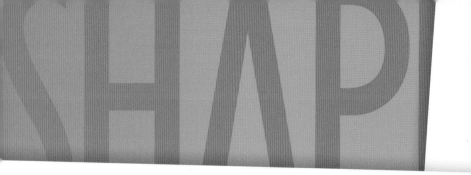

SHAPE

21100 Erwin Street,
Woodland Hills, California 91367-3772
Telephone (818) 595-0593
Fax (818) 704-5734

Jan. 31, 1995
Zipora Einav
4429 North Parkway Ave. #305
Scottsdale, AZ 85251
(602) 970-1110

Dear Zipora,
My husband and I are still having dreams about your roasted
pepper soup! Of the hundreds of spas I've visited as travel
editor of Shape magazine, never in my life have I tasted such
incredibly delicious and healthful spa cuisine. It was so
gorgeous I almost hated to eat it--until I tasted it. Then, I
couldn't stop! In fact, Tom said he has never seen me eat so
much in one sitting! Yet when I got home from the weekend
stay, my clothes felt looser than ever.
     As for you, Zipora, you are so warm and friendly and so
knowledgeable about cooking that I think you should write a
cookbook--or, even better, get those folks in Phoenix to give
you your own live television cooking show. I'm sure that with
your incredible personality and teaching skills, you'd be the
star of the Southwestern culinary world in about a week.
     Both of us can't wait to see you again in March and
sample more of your cooking! Thanks so much for the invitation
to your home. We'll be there with mucho grande appetites.
     I'll let you know as soon as I know about the Spa Food
piece. Generally, both Shape and Living Fit run a story focusing on three wonderful spa chefs once a year. Know that you'll
be a big part of both of them. I do a lot of freelance writing
as well, so let's see what I can cook up.
     Until we meet again, keep your pantry stocked, your pep-
pers roasted and may God bless you!

     Much love,

     Carole

     Carole Jacobs
     Articles/Adventure Travel Editor
     Shape Magazine

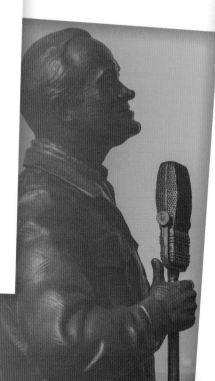

oyed her to prepare

a part of, for the duration

e who is familiar with the

is in good health, good

t a Chef who enjoys the

ransforms each bag of

o is healthy beyond

s on time and strives for

re than she is the

y.

sitation in answering any

t 9, 2000

om It May Concern:

Einav, know as Chef Zipora, is currently employed

vices were acquired due to the recording of my fourt

cess as present.

me of looking for a chef, it was important to find a per

nds the creative process, which Zipora is extremely se

as a household and as a production team enjoyed delici

lways unbelievably light and nutritious. In the time she

a repeated meal; her artistry as a chef is unsurpassed by

e is constantly preparing new concoctions that are indeed

rofessional and sensitive to an individuals needs. With a

of this album, it is important that I am of the highest leve

in every way Zipora has seen to it that I reach this goal.

free to contact my assistant Libby Murray at 310-275-4226

e no hesitation in answering any questions you may have.

ely,

Ritz Paris

ATTESTATION

Fait à Paris, le 22 février 2000

Je soussigné Monsieur Maurice GUILLOUET, Directeur des Cuisines de l'Hôtel Ritz, 15 place Vendôme à Paris 75001, atteste par la présente que Madame Zipora Einan a travaillé dans nos cuisines du vendredi 18 février au mercredi 23 février 2000 pendant son séjour à l'hôtel.

Elle a fait preuve de qualités personnelles et professionnelles appréciables dans l'accomplissement des tâches qui lui ont été confiées.

En foi de quoi, cette attestation est délivrée pour faire valoir ce que de droit.

Maurice GUILOUET
Directeur des Cuisines

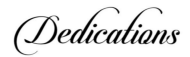

Dedications

TO MY SONS, David Einav and Rani Einav, for giving me the ultimate joy in life.

To my beautiful daughter-in-law, Scarlet, for your endless kindness and patience in helping me master my new iPad and overcome many computer challenges. The love and support that you and David give me unconditionally, along with my sweet grand-puppies, Lucy and Lucas, is the highlight of my days and keeps me smiling and laughing!

To my brother, Yoram, and my sister, Shosh, and brother-in-law, Shaul, for your unwavering love and support, and inspiring me to reach my dreams.

I also dedicate this book in memory of my mother, Yohevet, and my father, Yuhooda, for instilling in me the importance of generosity, warmth, and kindness toward all people.

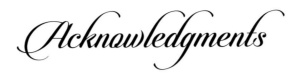

Acknowledgments

MANY TALENTED AND dedicated people helped make this book possible. I am so grateful to everyone for creating a beautiful book that exemplifies my passion for cooking, music, and caring for people. The pages come alive with many of my life's special moments, amazing culinary and travel experiences, and important life lessons.

To my wonderfully supportive business partner and friend, Jennifer Markson, thank you for dusting off my original manuscript and giving it new life. You brought together a great team to make this project an overwhelming success.

Thank you to David Welday and your gifted group of writers, designers, and project managers at HigherLife Publishing and Marketing; Andy Butcher, Will Hadley, and Michelle Buckley.

Thank you to Todd Moen and Leif Johnson at Interactive Apparel for making my book the first to include your company's new interactive technology. These new features greatly enhance my stories, making them colorful and lively while providing the reader with more information and a heightened entertainment value.

I had the great pleasure of working side by side with two talented and internationally recognized television and movie score composers, Neil Argo and Peter Vamos. I can't express in words the extent of my gratitude for the beautiful original music CDs you both created for this project.

To David Cogan, founder of Eliances. Thank you for creating an amazing support network of professionals in the Phoenix area, many of whom I can now call friends. I have never met so many extraordinary people as I have each week at the Eliances meetings.

Christine Jeffries, thank you for sharing your angelic voice on the Mozart children's CD and participating in filming my special "virtual" dinner for this book. To you and Kim Minert, I relish our friendship and it has been a joy to get to know you both. Your helping me network with new people through Eliances has been invaluable to my continued success.

To photographer Christopher Barr and production manager Jane Janssen, you both went above and beyond scouting out locations and finding the perfect spot to shoot the book cover images. You are an outstanding team, your creativity is limitless, and the artistic value of the photos is incredible!

Thank you to Lylah and Michael Ledner at The Simple Farm in Scottsdale, Arizona, for providing the perfect outdoor setting for Christopher Barr to capture beautiful images surrounded by nature's best.

To Dan Watts and your son, Chase, with NextWorld Media, you were both a pleasure to work with filming the "virtual" dinner and promotional video for my book. Your vision of the project, attention to detail, and storytelling ability is truly amazing and brought my book to life!

To Melissa Goodwin at AllState Appliances in Scottsdale, Arizona, I am grateful for your support and generosity in opening your lovely kitchen showroom area for me to film my recipe videos with NORMSCAR Video Productions.

To my food photographer, Rick Gayle, and food stylist, Kim Krejca, you managed to capture mouthwatering images of my food creations. Everyone who has seen the photos wants to pick the food up off the page and put it in their mouth. You are a pleasure to work with!

Reid Price, it was such a pleasure working with you to create a beautiful website. Your talent and work ethic are unmatched and well beyond your years! I wish you continued success in your new career. Many thanks also to Miranda Gilbert at Girl Geek Communications and Laura Bailey at Pen and Light Creative. Your proficiency with web design and establishing the new blog and online commerce capability has been instrumental to our success.

To Darcie Rowan and Heather Huzovic at Darcie Rowan PR agency, your expertise in book marketing and publicity has been an invaluable contribution. It is a pleasure working with both of you!

To Christian Paier, who placed me as private chef for Bob and Dolores Hope. Thank you for giving me the opportunity that jump-started my career and opened the door for other celebrities to hire me.

To my new friend Lulu, I can't thank you enough for your steadfast patience, support, and encouragement that always lift my spirit. Your wardrobe selections and makeup consultation made the photographs and video project a great success.

To my longtime friend Gisele Velos, you have always been there to support me and ready to say "yes" whenever I asked for help. I can't ever thank you enough!

Thank you to our fabulous attorneys who helped form Chef Zipora Enterprise: Barbara Luther, patent attorney, and Jeana Morrissey, business attorney. We truly appreciate your sound advice and direction. You made the process easy and enjoyable!

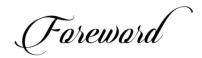

Foreword

Marrying Music and Cuisine for a Rich Life

WHEN SHAKESPEARE WROTE of music as "the food of love" in *Twelfth Night*, he hinted at what can be the profound, almost mystical connection between what we eat and what we hear. So perhaps it should not be surprising that some of the world's most gifted musicians have also been connoisseurs of fine cuisine.

Over the centuries, many composers have enjoyed the preparation and taste and combinations of different kinds of foods. They understood the way taste and texture could be intertwined, as they might weave together the different elements of a fine musical composition.

Everyone has heard of the four main food groups, but did you know that an orchestra has four principal instrument groupings? Woodwinds, brass, strings, and percussion can be combined with endless variations—just as can be elements of dairy, meat, fruits and vegetables, and grains.

Composers such as Vivaldi knew this; it's said that he enjoyed composing during his preparation of meals. Rossini was also well-known not only for his musical contributions but his culinary ones: among the dishes named after him are Tournedos Rossini, Eggs Rossini, and Pasta Rossini. One of his philosophies of the culinary and music world that he shared with friends was this observation:

"I know of no more admirable occupation than eating, that is really eating. Appetite is for the stomach what love is for the heart. The stomach is the conductor, who rules the grand orchestra of our passions, and rouses it to action."

Being familiar with the long-intertwined history of music and food, I was thrilled to be introduced to Chef Zipora, someone I found to be not only held in high esteem in culinary circles as an outstanding, world-class chef, but with an amazing sensibility for music and a special understanding of how music and cuisine are—or can be—reflections of each other.

When I was invited to work with her on a project bringing those two worlds together, I learned more of the unique way in which she sees cuisine as food/nutrition for the body and music as food/nutrition for the soul—each with limitless possibilities for color and taste combinations.

It was a great delight to create and produce an original piece celebrating this connection, for her website, in which I sought to blend original music stylings, with one theme running through different cultures of the world. Later I was pleased to have the opportunity to work with her further on creating classical music CDs for adults and children that seek to enhance food preparation and enjoyment.

Much has been written about how classical music can improve health and well-being. Sharing her professional and personal experiences in this fascinating book, Chef Zipora reveals more of all she has discovered about how we can experience life in all its best health and richness, and the part music can—truly—play in that discovery.

I believe the following pages will stir your appetite to taste for yourself.

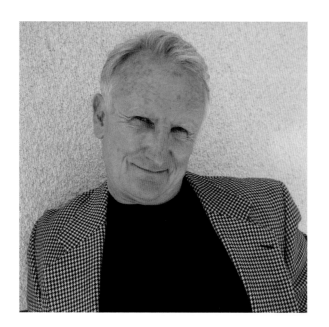

Neil Argo

Film and television composer, best known for his work on shows such as the new *Dynasty* series, *Beverly Hills 90210*, *MacGyver*, *Melrose Place*, (The New) *Mission Impossible*, and *Wild America*.

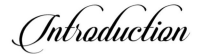

Introduction

My Recipe for a Better World

THEY SAY THAT an army marches on its stomach—that soldiers can fight only as well as they have been fed. I know this to be true from my own time wearing military fatigues and carrying a gun while fulfilling my mandatory service in the Israeli army.

But I have since learned while donning a different uniform and holding a different tool—a chef's jacket and a kitchen knife—that what is true for the battlefield is also true for the stage and the movie set. Musicians sing and play on their stomachs, while movie stars act on theirs.

It really does take a small army of people working behind the scenes to ensure that an artist or actor is at their best when they are in the spotlight or in front of the camera. And one of the most pivotal and personal roles is that played by the star's private chef.

After all, we are responsible for ensuring the performer looks and feels their best and is well-fueled for their demanding work. Whether it's a world concert tour or a blockbuster movie set, the success of a multi-million-dollar enterprise—and the livelihoods of countless people—depend on how well a private chef cares for their client's tummy.

That is quite a responsibility, as you might imagine. It's one that has taken me around the world, preparing gourmet meals alongside chefs from the finest luxury hotel kitchens— the Ritz in Paris, Claridge's in London, and the Imperial Hotel in Beijing—to Michelin-starred restaurants.

Along the way I have spoon-fed soup to an A-List singer, served afternoon tea to world-class musicians, and orchestrated many Hollywood dinners. Those who have dined on my food include social media star Kris Jenner; actors Robert Wagner, Jack Nicholson, Scarlett Johansson; and dozens of Hollywood executives and business people whose names don't make the gossip columns, but whose bank accounts and lifestyles rival those that do. My meals have been scarfed down in movie and television studios and savored under a starry Tuscan sky.

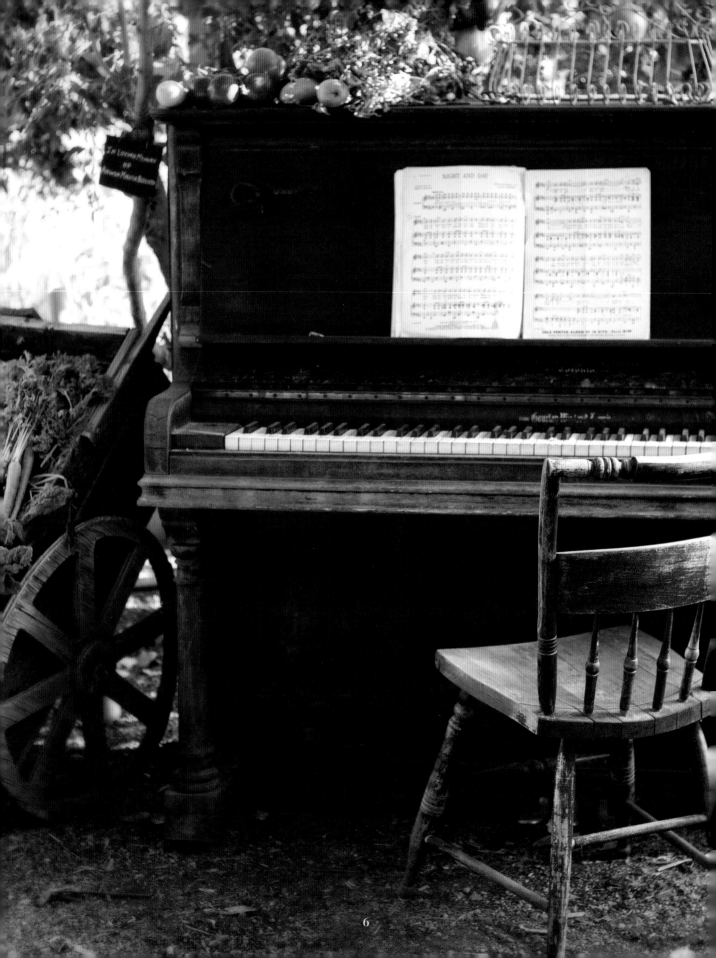

Because eating is such an intimate experience, I have seen celebrities in some of their most vulnerable moments, away from the bright lights. One thing I have learned about the rich and famous is that while they may have a lot more money than the rest of us, they aren't really that different.

They have many of the same joys and struggles, good days and bad. Some have shared stories of personal hardship as they have sat and eaten one of their favorite meals, which I prepared. In such moments, I believe I had the privilege of nourishing them not only physically, but emotionally.

It has been very satisfying to play a small part in helping entertain millions by ensuring that artists and actors are able to perform at their best. But even more, I have enjoyed knowing that I have been able to personally care for people I have come to care about.

Music, the Magic Ingredient

We can all do the same. You don't need to have lots of money and the fanciest equipment to be able to help people discover health and harmony with food. Serving people food that enriches their whole person in body, mind, and spirit takes some intention and effort—and the use of a very special ingredient.

Having traveled so much with singers, I have seen the powerful way in which music can touch people deeply. I have watched artists move crowds, turning cheers into tears, somehow feeding their audiences' emotions and souls with their melodies. At the close of a concert, many people leave feeling like they have just enjoyed a great banquet.

Seeing this magic happen on stage night after night reminded me of how, from being young, music has always been an important part of my life, and set me on a journey of

You don't need to have lots of money and the fanciest equipment to be able to help people discover health and harmony with food.

exploration. If music could touch people and if food could nourish people, I wondered, what might happen if we brought the two together more intentionally? The answer, I have discovered, is a whole other dimension.

I've had the opportunity to share some of what I have learned about healthy living and eating in a number of television appearances—one of which ended in a food fight live on air with the band members I was traveling with.

Now, in sharing some of my stories and experiences—and favorite recipes—with readers, I want to pass along to a wider audience some of what I have learned about how you can enjoy a more delicious life, and help those you care about do the same.

Experiencing greater health and harmony with food isn't only personally satisfying—though it is that in good measure. I believe it also releases greater health and harmony into the wider world.

So much of the division and anger we see around us today comes from inside. When we are not happy with ourselves, we tend not to be happy with other people either. The result too often can be prejudice and hate. But when we are at peace with ourselves, we have peace to share with others.

I am not saying that eating well and helping others eat well will solve all the world's problems, but it's a good place to start. Here's my recipe for helping make a better world for us all.

MARIAH CAREY'S ROASTED RED AND YELLOW PEPPER SOUP

A taste test is an important part of a celebrity's selection process for choosing a private chef. This soup secured my place on Mariah's Rainbow world tour.

(Serves 4)

Ingredients

YELLOW PEPPER SOUP	RED PEPPER SOUP	SERRANO CREAM
1 Tablespoon Virgin Olive Oil	1 Tablespoon Virgin Olive Oil	3 Fresh Serrano Chilies or Jalapeños (seeded and finely chopped)
1 Tablespoon Butter	1 Tablespoon Butter	1 Garlic Clove (minced and mashed to a paste with 1/2 teaspoon salt)
6 Yellow Peppers	6 Red Peppers	1/2 cup Crème Fraîche (or Sour Cream)
2 Tablespoons Yellow Onion (finely diced)	2 Tablespoons Yellow Onion (finely diced)	
1 Medium Carrot (peeled and finely diced)	1 Medium Carrot (peeled and finely diced)	
1 Stick Celery (finely diced)	1 Stick Celery (finely diced)	
1/2 Teaspoon Dry Thyme	1/2 Teaspoon Dry Thyme	
Salt and Black Pepper	Salt and Black Pepper	
Pinch of Cayenne	Pinch of Cayenne	
1/4 Cup Heavy Cream (or Almond Milk)	1/4 Cup Heavy Cream (or Almond Milk)	
1/2 Teaspoon Fresh Lemon Juice	1/2 Teaspoon Fresh Lemon Juice	
1-1/2 Cups Vegetable Broth	1-1/2 Cups Vegetable Broth	

Instructions

Cooking note: Broil peppers in the oven OR for a smoky flavor cook over an open flame on gas stove-top.

1. Adjust tray in oven to 6 inches under broiler; preheat to high.

2. Arrange peppers on baking sheet.

3. Bake peppers until skin looks black; flip and continue baking until all sides are evenly black.

4. Turn off broiler and remove peppers; cover with plastic wrap for 5 minutes.

5. When peppers are cool enough to handle, remove skin and seeds from peppers (don't wash them or they will lose their flavor!); slice into strips and put to the side, still separating the red from the yellow.

6. Heat oil and butter in 2 separate pots. Add half amount of each of the onions, carrots, celery, salt, pepper, cayenne, and thyme. Bring to a simmer for 8-10 minutes.

7. Add the red and yellow peppers separately to each of the pots and mix well. Add half amount of the vegetable broth to each pot and simmer for another 10-12 minutes.

8. Taking turns, place red and yellow peppers in blender and mix separately to a puree; cover while blending. (For a finer soup, you can put the mixture through a fine strainer. Otherwise, leave it chunky.)

9. Place blended red and yellow peppers back in their respective pots on low heat. Add the cream (or almond milk), lemon juice, salt and pepper to taste.

10. To make the serrano cream: in a blender, mix together the chilies, garlic paste, and créme fraiche until the mixture is combined well. (Be careful not to over-blend.)

To serve: Pour the yellow and red pepper soups into separate measuring cups. Simultaneously, pour 2 cups of each into a soup bowl for serving. Decorate with a dollop of serrano cream.

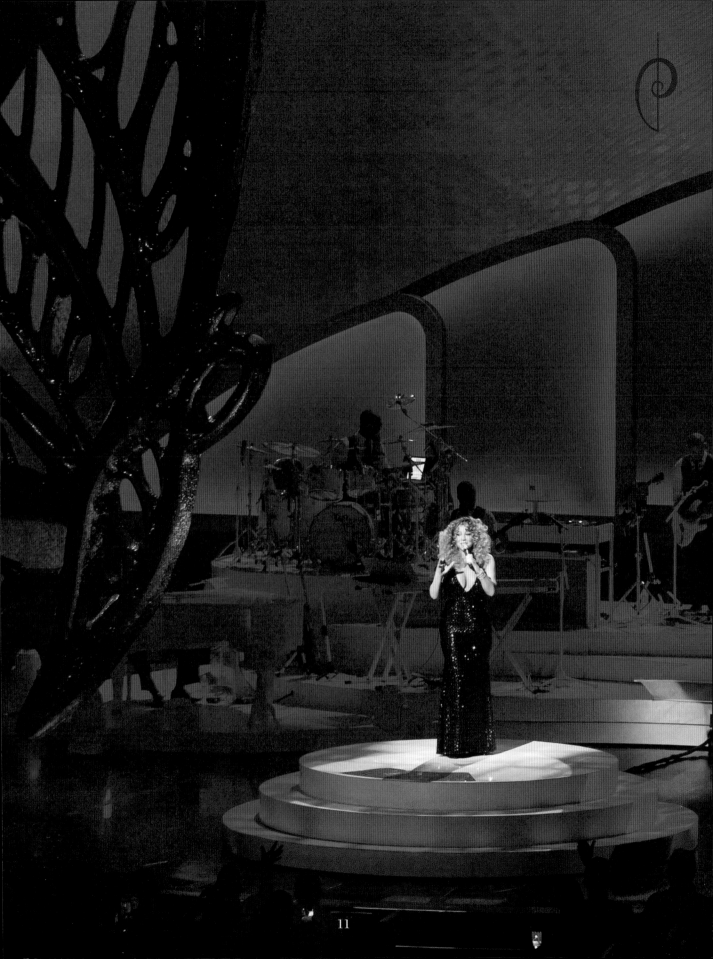

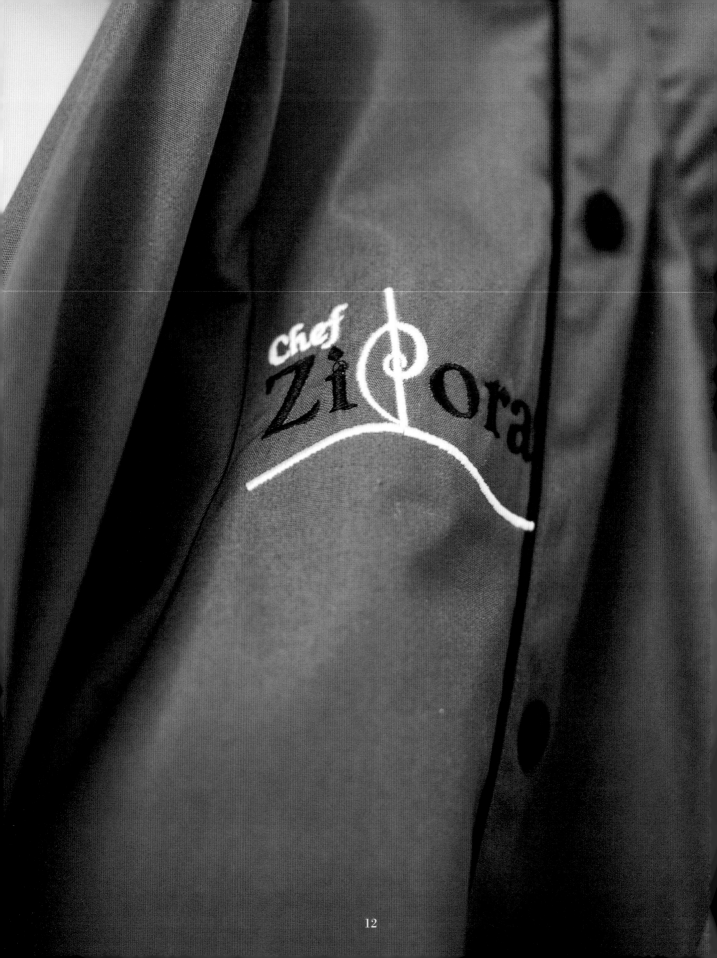

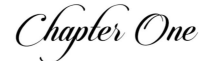

Chapter One

A Taste for Adventure, a Zest for Life

LIKE ANY CHEF, I am always glad to know that my food has been appreciated. Celebrity clients have come into the kitchen to thank me in person, or brought me into their dining room at the end of private meals I have catered to introduce me to their guests. That has been gratifying—and has often led to more business from people in attendance who asked for my card.

I have always been thankful for these small moments of gratitude. But there was one time when I squirmed—as thousands of people clapped and cheered.

It came during the couple of years I toured with The Kelly Family as their private chef. Comprising ten siblings who sang and played a wide range of instruments, this American-Irish family band was especially popular in Europe, touring in a big old double-decker bus and performing sell-out concerts in stadiums and other large venues.

I was excited to learn recently that several of the original band members have reformed The Kelly Family and are touring in Europe again after a break of many years. I'm hoping to have the opportunity to see them perform in their new show. It would be fun to catch up with them and recall some of our adventures together. Through the two years I worked with the band, I became a part of the extended family, not only preparing all their food but also dispensing words of comfort and encouragement whenever needed. Their mother had passed away, so in some ways I became something of a surrogate mom to them. I'd greet them with hugs when they came off stage after a show, telling them how well they had done, handing out towels and robes so they could wipe the sweat off and keep warm.

This wasn't one of my official responsibilities, but I saw it as part of caring for them as whole persons. My main job was to provide lunch, dinner before their evening show, and then something light for them after the performance. As you might imagine, that didn't leave me with a lot of down time.

However, on occasions I could take a short break during their performance. I never got tired of hearing them play, so I'd stand to the side of the stage to enjoy their music, or occasionally make my way down in front, with the rest of the audience.

That is where I was standing one night during a concert in Germany when one of them spotted me in the crowd. I am not sure how they saw me—I'm only 5 ft., 1 in. tall. Maybe I stood out because I still had my white chef's jacket on.

Anyway, the next thing I knew, between songs I was being summoned to join them on stage. Reluctantly I made my way through the crowd and around to the steps and up onto the stage, where the band introduced me, telling everyone how much they loved me, my food, and how well I looked after them.

All the applause was a little embarrassing, but it did remind me how I had first fallen in love with providing people with good food, many years before.

Seasoned With Obligation

I didn't discover how satisfying good food can be, physically and emotionally, until I was about eight years old. Growing up in Hadera, a small community between Haifa and Tel Aviv, on Israel's Mediterranean coast, I didn't look forward to family meal times.

Being together with my parents and two siblings was fine, but the food was another story. Though we lived on a small farm that produced beautiful fresh vegetables we sold in the grocery store my mother ran, she served heavy and often sweetened dishes from Eastern Europe.

Both Jewish, Mom and my father had met and married in Israel after fleeing Poland and Lithuania, respectively, before World War II. Sadly, many of our relatives who stayed behind died in Hitler's purge.

Settling in Israel before it achieved statehood, in 1948, my parents worked long hours to make a life for themselves as part of a small Zionist community. In addition to working hard, they were kind and generous. It wasn't unusual for them to come across people who had nowhere to live and invite them to stay with us for a while. They'd feed and house them without any charge.

Dad was employed overseeing road construction while Mom managed the grocery store.

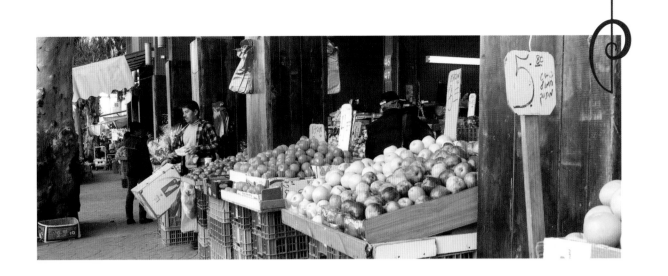

She did this in addition to running the household and being the main caregiver of three children, which meant she didn't have a lot of time or energy left for food preparation. I don't blame my mom for her weariness in any way, but it was clear that feeding us was just another chore.

Friday nights were the worst. This was when she would prepare Gefilte fish, a traditional dish for the weekly Shabbat dinner. Though my parents were not religious, they did observe some of the traditions of the Jewish calendar.

I loathed the taste of this stuffed fish, which Mom fixed with sugar in the East European tradition. I came up with all the excuses I could for not eating it: my throat hurt, my stomach was upset, I was already full, I was so tired. But my Mom wasn't stupid. She gave me increasingly smaller portions as time went by.

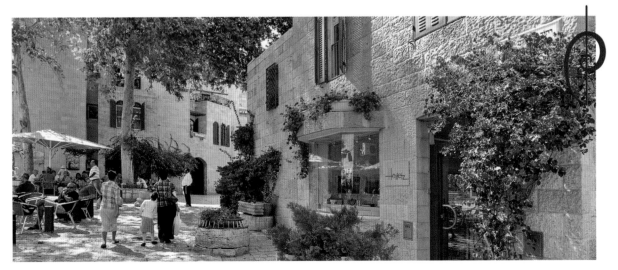

It would be years before I realized that it was her absence of interest in or enthusiasm for what my mom was doing in the kitchen which was the missing ingredient that made everything taste so bad to me. Some cooks ruin meals by over-salting everything. In my mother's case, it seemed like her meals were spoiled by a heavy seasoning of obligation.

There were a couple of exceptions. She could make a delicious dessert on occasions, and her tagine, a Moroccan-style stew, was quite delicious. But these treats were all too rare. As a result, I was quite skinny. Some people might even have considered me to be malnourished.

One way I was able to keep from starving was by going to get the fresh black bread we bought each morning from a nearby bakery. Still warm from the oven, it was so tasty that I would usually eat a good portion of one of the two loaves before I got back to the house.

At some stage, I discovered there were other things close to hand that could satisfy my appetite. We grew all sorts of vegetables and fruit in the fields and trees around our home: apples, apricots, avocados, carrots, cucumbers, mangoes, mushrooms, persimmon, and tomatoes. We also had a chicken coop and the geese, turkeys, and goats we owned all ran wild.

Whenever I wanted a fresh, tasty carrot or tomato, or an apple or pear, I could help myself by picking up one from the ground or plucking the ripest fruit from one of the trees. It was the juiciest treat you can image! On occasion, I would also take a freshly laid egg, crack the shell, and drink down the raw yolk and white. Delicious.

Trial and Error

In time, I experimented with all this readily available fresh food. I'd carefully layer pieces of the lettuce greens and arrange them with different vegetables on top, creating a salad on my plate so the colors sat well together and the different textures and shapes looked pleasing to my keen artistic eye. It made me happy to admire my new creations and eating them was so much more enjoyable.

My brother, Yoram, and my cousins Shoshana and Abraham noticed what I was doing in the kitchen. They started asking me to prepare some of my salads for them, which I did gladly. In a busy household, it was nice to hear words of affirmation.

Their appreciation made me feel warm and full inside, just like the fresh bread from the bakery. I didn't make the connection back then, but it was the first time I experienced giving and receiving love and affection through the preparing and sharing of food. I didn't realize this would become the driving passion of my life.

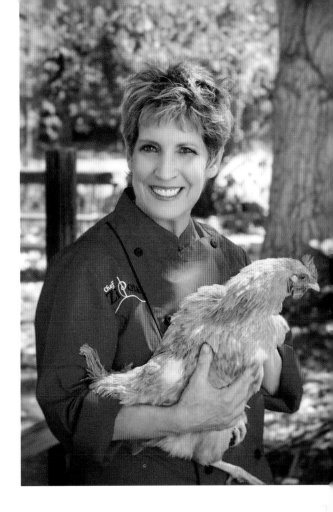

I had already learned that cooking can involve some trial and error, however. At the age of five or so, I had decided to help my mother with one of her meals.

Though we were not orthodox Jews, Mom sent our chickens to the shochet, the kosher butcher. He would butcher one and leave it on our kitchen counter. Mom would later put the chicken in a pressure cooker, to save preparation time.

Well, when I saw the chicken on the side there one day, back from the shochet and ready to be cooked, I decided that I would ease Mom's burden. I stuffed the bird into the pot just as it was—oblivious that it had not been cleaned or plucked.

Not knowing how long to let it cook, I decided after a while that it must surely be done. But I didn't know how to release the pressure from the pot, and the lid would not budge. Finally, I got my father's hammer and with a big swing knocked the lid off.

It spun away like a flying saucer, smashing through the sliding glass door and into the backyard. Thankfully, I was unharmed. But the chicken shot straight up into the air where, by force of the tremendous impact, it stuck to the ceiling.

Something of a cleanliness freak, my mom kept the glass of the sliding door so spotless that when she came home that evening she didn't notice right away that it was missing. Then she felt the breeze from the outdoors. Looking up, she saw the chicken still pasted to the ceiling, feathers and all. Fortunately, she could only look at me and laugh.

Meanwhile, I was making other discoveries that would weave into the way I nourished other people when I got older. With Yoram several years older than me, and my sister, another Shoshana in the family whom we called "Shosh," six years younger, we didn't play together much. And though I had some friends, I was often on my own.

...you can be alone without being lonely—just as you can feel alone in a crowded room...

But you can be alone without being lonely—just as you can feel alone in a crowded room—and I was quite happy with my own company for long periods of time. I had taught myself to read by the age of four or five, and would spend hours by myself in my room, with a book from my parents' extensive library.

Every Passover, we would have a thorough house-cleaning as part of the preparation and celebration. My job was to climb a ladder and clean all the bookshelves. The only problem was that I'd often stop to pull out a book I hadn't read, and find myself so engrossed that I would forget about the dusting. That did not make me very popular with Yoram when he was sent to see how I was getting on.

Still, to this day I'm grateful for the love of reading I developed at an early age, which has enabled me to expand my understanding of food, health, and nutrition by doing my own studying.

Learning to Leap

Around the same time that I developed a passion for books, I also began to explore music. I am not sure where this interest came from. Yoram was quite musical, learning to play the trumpet, but we didn't listen to a lot of music in the house. We would play the radio sometimes, but Mom wanted it switched off when she came home. She'd had enough noise from being in the store all day long.

However it developed, my love of music became clear to my parents and for one of my birthdays they bought me a record player. I was thrilled. Sitting in my room with a book, I'd listen to records endlessly.

Though I was young, I was not particularly drawn to popular music. I found myself being tugged by classical recordings—first Bach and then others such as Vivaldi and Handel. In time I discovered opera, getting swept up in works such as Puccini's *Madame Butterfly*. Any money I received as gifts or earned for doing chores or helping out at the store would go to buying new LPs from the record store.

Rather than playing with friends, I would sit alone in my room for hours, getting lost in the sound around me. Whatever my mood, the music could meet me there—happy, sad, lonely. I felt calm, peaceful, joyful, resting in the melodies and sweep of the music. This was as close to a religious experience as I would have.

It would be many years before I put together all those elements from my childhood in a way that touched other people's lives. Just as the right preparation is an important dimension of a wonderful meal, I had to go through a bunch of life experiences that brought me to the right time and place.

They included mandatory service in the Israeli army, two years for women and three for men. I learned a lot during the time I served in military intelligence, including discipline, determination, independence, how to think on your feet and outside the box, and teamwork.

I also discovered what it takes to overcome fear—a lesson that came the hard way. As part of a training exercise they split up a group of us taking a leadership course, escorting half to the top of a four-story building. The others were down below, holding out a stretched army blanket onto which we had to jump.

If we didn't go voluntarily, we were told, we would be pushed.

"Right, who wants to go first?" one of the leaders asked.

I immediately raised my hand. "I'll do it."

But I made a big mistake. When I got to the edge of the roof, I did the one thing the instructors had warned us not to: I looked down. In an instant, my mind told me to step away.

Everybody else in the group then took their turns to jump while I waited, ashamed of backing down. Finally only I remained. With a deep breath I stepped forward and fell to the blanket.

From that day on, I vowed to myself that I would never again let fear hold me back from stepping off the edge.

A Whole New World

The determination that came from my moment on the ledge fueled my decision to immigrate to America. After years focused on raising two boys, and the end of my marriage, I decided I wanted to make a new start for us. To be sure of getting one of the limited number of visas, I waited outside the United States Embassy in Tel Aviv, sleeping on the ground overnight to be first in line the next morning.

I was undaunted by the fact that I didn't speak a word of English when I landed in Los Angeles, where I was going to stay for a while with Yoram and his wife, who had settled there. Call it a mix of craziness and confidence, but it paid off—though not without some amusing moments.

One of my favorite items of clothing was a brightly designed T-shirt with English script, which I'd bought back in Israel. I thought wearing it would help me fit in. When everybody smiled and laughed when I met them, I just assumed that all Americans were friendly and kind—until I was told that the T-shirt read, "Smile if you got screwed today."

After several months, and with a better grasp of the language, I moved to Phoenix at the invitation of some new friends. Looking to get financially secure enough to bring my sons over, I took whatever work I could find, including cleaning houses.

When I cooked and invited friends over, some of them asked if I would prepare something special for birthday parties or other events they were holding. Encouraged by this new interest in my cooking, when some of my housecleaning clients asked me to help tidy up before or after events, I would tell them that I could cater, as well.

Bit by bit word got around, and over time I began to build up quite a successful little business, Zipora Catering. In addition to providing food for private events, I got some corporate clients, and started delivering lunches to businesses.

Almost before I knew it, I was leasing space in a commercial kitchen to handle everything, with several employees. Life was good. My boys were with me now, and I was doing what I loved and getting paid for it.

A few years later, an old friend contacted me. She and her husband had moved to LA, and they invited me to stay with them and see whether I might find work there. The city always reminded me of my childhood near the ocean. As much as I enjoyed living in Arizona, I missed the greenery I had grown up around on the Israeli coast.

Something in my gut told me to jump off again. Doing so set off a fast-moving chain of events that opened up a whole new world to me.

Within a few months I had sold my business in Phoenix and gone west. A couple of days before heading out to LA, I visited a friend who was a psychic. She told me that I was going to be very successful, that I would work with celebrities and travel the world.

She also told me she was going to connect me with one of her phone clients. This woman lived in Los Angeles and had been the private chef to one of Hollywood's biggest A-List couples. Maybe she could help connect me with some clients.

I hadn't been thinking about working with show business people, but I welcomed the introduction that could lead to some income. On my first day in Los Angeles I met this friend-of-a-friend for dinner. We hit it off, and she told me of a gentleman she knew, named Chris, who was opening a new chef agency. Apparently there was a big market in Los Angeles for private chefs, not only among those in the entertainment industry but also in other high-net-worth circles.

When Chris and I met the following morning, he told me his agency was so new that he didn't even have business cards printed yet. Clearly, he was a newcomer to this type of catering, so I was honest with him about my own experience.

"Look, I'm self-taught," I said, telling him about my passion for helping others live healthier lives because of what they ate and how that made them feel. I told him how quickly my catering business had grown in Phoenix, and shared some of the testimonials from satisfied clients.

"I can't make any promises," he said as we finished our meeting. "But I will keep you in mind. The phone can ring at any time."

Mine did a little later the same day. It was Chris. Someone had called with an opening.

And that was how, on my third day in Los Angeles, I found myself on Bob Hope's doorstep.

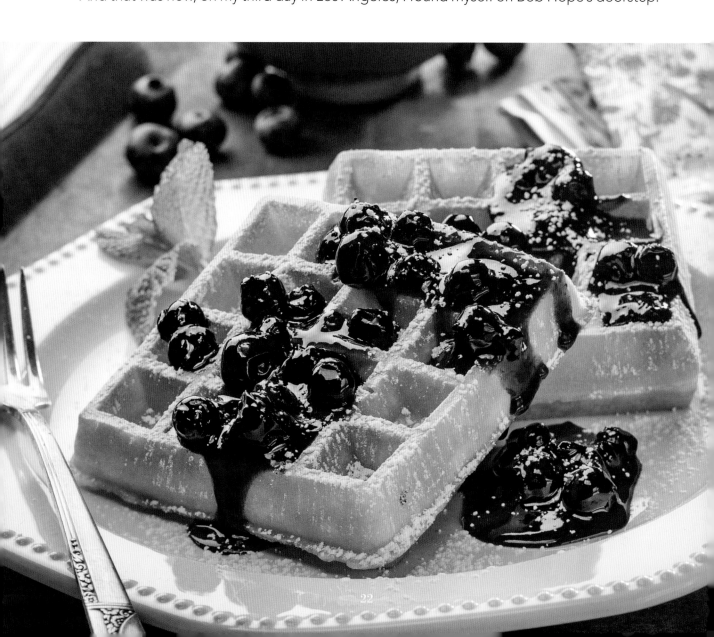

THE KELLY FAMILY'S WAFFLES WITH BLUEBERRY SAUCE

We were staying at a beautiful luxury hotel in Beijing, where one of the chefs was curious about what I was making for the band's Sunday brunch. He wanted to know how to cook an American brunch, so I shared my waffles recipe with him—and in return, he taught me how to make authentic Chinese sauces.

(Serves 4)

Ingredients

WAFFLES

2 Cups All-Purpose Flour

4 Teaspoons Baking Powder

2 Tablespoons Sugar

2 Eggs (at room temperature)

1-½ Cups Whole Milk (warm)

2 Tablespoons Melted Butter

1 Teaspoon Vanilla Extract

BLUEBERRY SAUCE

1-½ Cups Blueberries

2-3 Tablespoons Honey

½ Cup Fresh Orange Juice

1 Tablespoon Cornstarch

Instructions

WAFFLES

1. Separate egg yolks from the whites.

2. Mix flour, salt, baking powder, and sugar.

3. Using a hand mixer or blender, mix the egg whites until soft peaks form.

4. Preheat waffle iron.

5. In a bowl, combine eggs, milk, butter, and vanilla.

6. Mix in the dry ingredients and then gently blend in the egg whites (don't over-mix!).

7. Using a large spoon, pour batter onto the waffle iron and cook to a golden brown.

BLUEBERRY SAUCE

1. In a saucepan over medium heat, mix 1-½ cups blueberries, honey, and ¼ cup orange juice; bring to a boil.

2. Mix remaining orange juice and cornstarch in a bowl; add to the blueberry mixture.

3. Stir constantly until thickened.

4. Pour over the waffles.

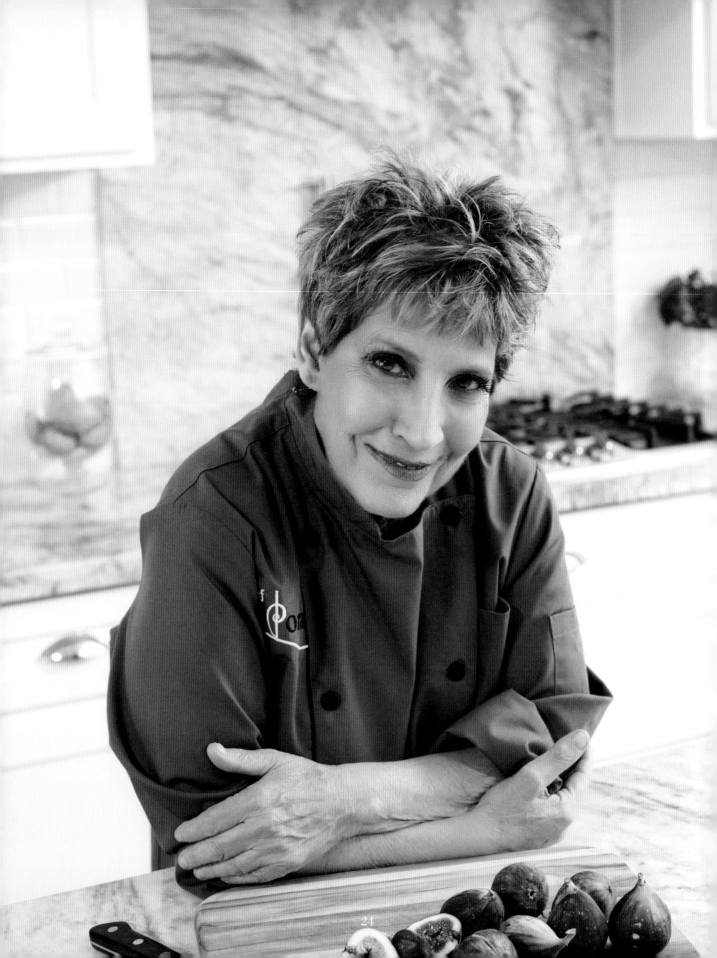

24

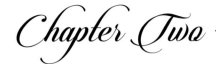
The Kitchen Is the Heart of Your Home

AN ESSENTIAL PART of healthy eating is using the right ingredients, of course. But it doesn't start there. For me, the foundation is not what foods you work with, but where and how you work with them.

I have been fortunate during my career to have enjoyed free access to some of the most amazing kitchens in the world, from multi-million-dollar celebrity homes fitted out with every piece of equipment and gadget available to the best of luxury hotels.

But I have learned that's not enough if you want to nourish people with your food. You can have the finest setting, but if the atmosphere of the kitchen isn't right you won't be able to serve from your heart. It's like having a high-performance car and trying to run it on cheap gas.

I believe the kitchen is the most important room in a home—it's the engine that drives everywhere and everything else. And I'm not just saying that because I'm a chef.

Have you noticed how people love to gather in the kitchen, whether they are eating or not? Think of parties you've been to. How often was it the place where guests tended to gravitate? With all those people there, you might expect to have found some wonderful treats being handed out, but often there was nothing but people standing around talking. So why in the kitchen?

It's because the kitchen plays a unique role within the home and in our lives. In *Relish: An Adventure in Food, Style, and Everyday Fun,* Daphne Oz, co-host of ABC's *The Chew,* writes, "The kitchen is the most basic source of creativity in a home." I agree. It's also our source of survival and nourishment. It's like the heart of the home, producing sustenance that circulates throughout the rest of our lives.

I had sensed that from when I was a little girl. Even though I hadn't enjoyed much of what my mother had prepared while in the kitchen, I had been drawn to the place because it was the hub of the home. I'd offer to help clean the dishes so I could be around there.

When I was growing up in Israel it was well known that the former Prime Minister, Golda Meir, Israel's only woman leader, used to hold her cabinet meetings in the kitchen of her official residence. She apparently felt she could get more done there.

Just as a body can only be as healthy as the heart that beats within it, so a healthy kitchen is essential to a life-giving home. But what is a healthy kitchen? Most people understand the importance of cleanliness, but only think about it on a very superficial level: wipe the counters and shelves, disinfect the sink, self-clean the oven and you're ready to go, right?

Those are all good things, but they are only dealing with the surface.

We've all been places where we just know the past lingers, haven't we? We sense something in the air—maybe great love, or perhaps immense sadness. That feeling is never more true

---

Most kitchens may have vents to extract bad odors, but the bad vibes can remain.

---

than when we are in a kitchen, where we do a lot of our living, and it isn't always pretty. We laugh and cry, we bicker and make up. Most kitchens may have vents to extract bad odors, but the bad vibes can remain.

I don't believe in ghosts, but I am sure that sometimes we can sense the residual energy of people that stagnates and collects in places. That's why one person's home might feel comfortable while another's home, though it is nicely furnished, might have you itching to escape. It's not because of the drapes, carpets, and color scheme; it's the energy in the air.

The Worst Toxins

We hear a lot in the news about global warming and other effects of toxicity on our living. But there's nothing more noxious than human toxicity. While it's true that all objects possess and project energy we're capable of feeling, without a doubt the most dominant energy is that of people.

Working in a contaminated kitchen is like preparing food beside someone working with poisonous chemicals. You have clean food in a dirty environment. Why put your heart into making wonderfully nutritious food, when all the time it's being tainted by stale and negative energy?

As a society, we are more aware of the dangerous toxins being released in our world through industries. But we are less conscious that we are releasing toxins through individuals, too—poisonous emotions such as hate, rage, envy and, perhaps the biggest one of all, indifference.

When I walk into someone's kitchen for the first time, I can immediately learn quite a bit about them—probably more than some would want me to know. I can read the space like a detective searching for clues at the scene of a crime. Messy silverware drawers usually mean they aren't very organized. Old food left in the refrigerator or cupboards suggests stagnation and neglect. Dishes piled in the sink expose a tendency toward procrastination.

The worst kitchen in Hollywood I ever worked in belonged to a major entertainment executive who lived in a sprawling multi-million-dollar mansion. It was decorated with the most extravagant, plush furniture and window treatments, with "extras" that featured a built-in bowling alley, and a fifty-person staff.

While this may sound inviting, the kitchen might as well have been a morgue. It occupied a huge space—as big as some houses. If you wanted to get in shape, you could roller skate back and forth from one end to the other and get a good workout. Like the rest of the house, every appliance and tool in the kitchen was of the high-priced variety, but that didn't help. The area was cold, without character, and totally lifeless. A dead zone.

It seemed like whoever had created this kitchen had no intention of using it. When they brought me in to cook, I could barely function. Two assistants stood over me while I tried to prepare a meal. They wouldn't let me bring anything. As soon as I asked where a certain ingredient might be found, they scurried away to retrieve it for me. The moment I put down a knife, they'd scoop it up for washing.

You'd think with so much help that I would have loved working there. But I couldn't stop looking at my watch. When would it be time to go home? How much longer did I have to stay?

This was very strange for me because I always loved cooking. Usually I enjoyed myself so much that I forgot about time and lost myself in the act of food preparation. This kitchen made me continuously aware of time and my desire to leave.

After cooking a few dinners there I refused to go back. Though I was giving up good money, I felt an overwhelming sense of relief. Later I learned that although the cooking position paid top dollar, they could never keep it filled. I wasn't the only one who couldn't stand to prepare meals in that kitchen.

Nor am I alone in recognizing the importance of a positive environment when preparing food. In *Relish*, Oz writes a good kitchen is essential for her "to feel inspired to prepare the foods that will keep me and mine feeling happy and energized all week long."

One of the celebrity kitchens I most enjoyed working in was that of actor Pierce Brosnan and his wife, Keely Shaye Smith. Overlooking the beautiful Pacific Ocean, the space invited you in and pulsated with life. It wasn't just because it was well-appointed. There was such a harmonious feeling, as if a symphony was going on and you were sitting right in the middle of it. I liked being there so much that I didn't want to go home at the end of the day.

Considering the working conditions, it was no surprise that Pierce and Keely loved the food I prepared for them in their kitchen. They told me all the time how great what I prepared for them tasted. Pierce especially enjoyed my roasted squash soup with apples, and Keely asked my advice for a cookbook she was working on. They were lovely, down-to-earth people, and their kind and generous nature permeated their kitchen with a welcoming atmosphere.

Clearing the Air

Another time, I was hired to cook for a famous movie actress. I was looking forward to working with her, but when I walked into her kitchen the energy was so chaotic that I could barely focus. My thoughts were scattered. A meal that would typically take an hour to prepare required twice the time.

I discovered she never cooked for herself on a regular basis. She was always on the run, grabbing a quick bite here or there. Her kitchen was more like a pit-stop at a race track than a place for nourishment and refreshment. This hectic energy hung in the air. No wonder I felt so scattered.

I told her I needed to harmonize her kitchen if I was going to keep working there. I explained this was sort of like a spring-cleaning, clearing out the "cobwebs" of the past and refreshing the space.

It was a practice that had been born in a cave, believe it or not. Let me explain.

One of the first things you learn when you are on the road with a rock band is to be flexible. With a different venue almost every day, you never know quite what circumstances you will have to deal with.

Before I set out on a European tour with The Kelly Family, I had designed my own state-of-the-art mobile kitchen. It traveled in a set of flight cases, like their band instruments, and was better equipped than many restaurants. Regardless of where I found myself on our travels, I knew I had the equipment in hand that I would need to prepare the band's daily meals.

But even this preparedness was tested when we arrived in Pula, a resort town on the Croatian coast, across the Adriatic Sea from Italy. Pula was beautiful, like an undiscovered paradise. The sea was the bluest I'd ever seen. And, oh my, the fresh fruit: juicy watermelon, fresh and crisp as an apple, and plump figs as big as my fist. Coming from Israel, the land of such amazing fruits, I was impressed. I thought we had arrived at the Garden of Eden, only better because it had beautiful beaches too.

Then the tour manager showed me where my kitchen was going to be set up. My heart hit the floor. I'd gone from paradise to hell.

The concert was to take place in Pula's ancient Roman amphitheater. Now this was a fantastic place to put on a show, for sure. But as the site of cruel gladiator games, steeped in two thousand years of violent history, it was hardly an ideal cooking environment.

Heightening the challenging nature of my task was the space I was given in which to set up my mobile kitchen—in an actual cave at the back of the venue.

While the roadies unloaded my kitchen gear, I was pulling my hair out wondering what to do. Tours run on a tight schedule, and I did not have much time to make the most of this challenging situation.

The cave was so small that my kitchen equipment barely fit in it. The ceiling was low, while some cement tiles covered the floor. A coat of paint had been applied to the walls in a half-hearted attempt to brighten things up. Stuffy and airless, it wasn't dirty and it wasn't clean. It was characterless and unwelcoming. I could feel everything that had happened there—the conflict, the violence.

The whole place brought out almost an allergic reaction in me. I kept walking in and out, but I didn't want to unpack the kitchen equipment. I looked at my watch and knew I had to get started. I needed to shop at the local market and then a meal to prepare for the band before showtime.

I decided I would have to transform the cave myself. Quickly I headed to the market with the personal assistant assigned to me, someone who spoke the language and knew the currency. I bought some watermelon and figs to fortify myself and other fresh fruit and vegetables for cooking. Then I paid for flowers, candles, and incense.

Back at the cave, I set out my flowers, lit my candles, and burned the incense. I threw salt into each of the corners as a symbolic cleansing. Next I reached for my African drum. I traveled with it because I liked to play after work to relax. I had never formally learned to play a musical instrument, but my years of soaking in classical music had somehow given me a sense and a feel for rhythm.

As a child, I'd wandered into an empty music room at the end of the school day, one time, and sat at the piano picking out notes and simple melodies by ear. Swept up in the wonder of creating even elementary music, I lost all track of time before realizing I would be late getting home and rushing back to ask Mom if I could have piano lessons.

I swallowed my disappointment when she said no. But that sense of yearning to not just savor music, but somehow become part of it, never went away. I found myself instinctively tapping out rhythms to whatever I was listening to, like you would on a drum. Years later, I'd realize that the piano, of course, was also a percussion instrument.

Looking back, I sometimes wonder if I had been encouraged more as a child, whether I might have pursued music more seriously. As it was, music was just something that I needed in my life in some way, as I developed my gifts in the kitchen. As I got older, I taught myself to play the harmonica and I also learned to play the drums. My nephew, who is a talented musician, always comments on my natural sense of rhythm when he lets me play around on his drum set. With his help, I had picked out the African drum that became part of my traveling equipment.

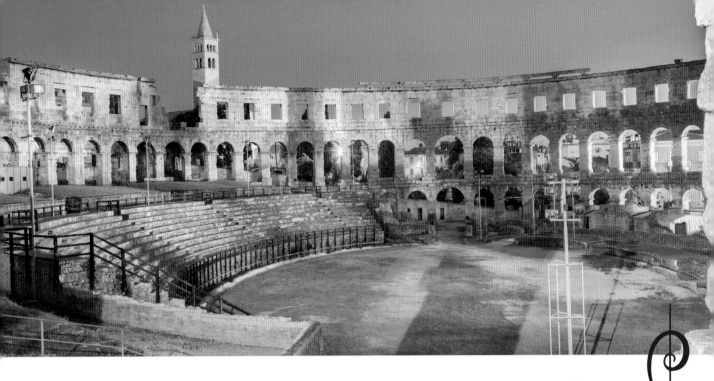

Pulling it out in that Pula cave, I hit it very hard. I wanted to take out my frustrations about my makeshift kitchen, but then I found something magical starting to happen. It was like a cork popping out of a champagne bottle. Something in that cave gave way.

The unwelcoming energy dissolved and a sweet feeling came over the place—calm and inviting. I felt comfortable, like I wanted to stay there, like I was at home. Before I hadn't wanted to stay in the cave; now I didn't want to leave. I played some lively Balkan folk music on my portable CD player, opened my equipment cases, and got to work.

A funny thing happened. People started finding reasons to come into the cave and see me. They began bringing me CDs to play, asking me questions, checking to see how I was doing—any excuse to be in there with me, it seemed.

This was a cramped space, however, and I needed to get a lot done in a short period of time. I had to kick people out just to work. As soon as I shooed one person away, someone else came in. The cave that I couldn't stand to walk into had become the place to gather.

Even The Kelly Family band members came in, which surprised me. Normally, they were busy with soundchecks or resting before going on stage. During the tour I'd become very close with all the family, and I loved cooking for them, but to be sure to have their food ready in time I had to kick them out too.

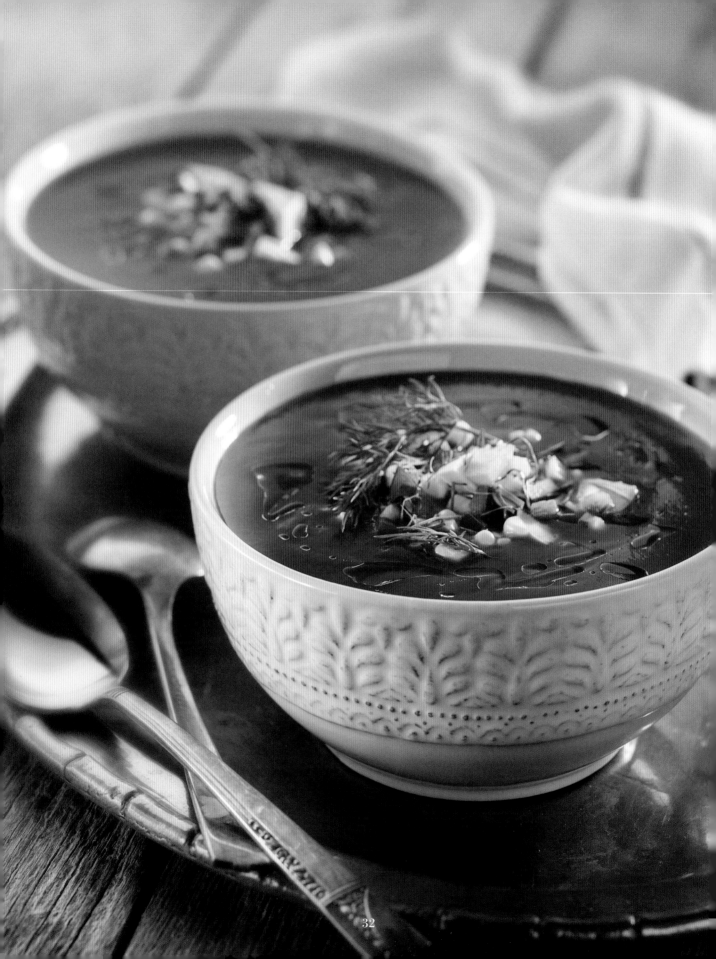

PIERCE BROSNAN'S HEIRLOOM TOMATO SOUP WITH SUCCOTASH

I loved cooking for the former "James Bond - 007" Pierce Brosnan and his wife, Keely Shaye Smith. They especially enjoyed the sense of farm-freshness I often try to capture in my recipes.

(Serves 4)

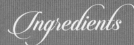

Ingredients

SOUP

6 Heirloom Tomatoes (any color)

1 Tablespoon Sherry Vinegar

2 Tablespoons Extra Virgin Olive Oil

1 Tablespoon Fresh Lemon Juice

Salt and Pepper to taste

SUCCOTASH

1-2 Garlic Cloves

½ Medium Sweet Onion

1 Cup Green Peas

½ Cup Fava Beans

1 Cup Corn Kernels

1 Tablespoon Fresh Lemon Juice

Chive Flowers or Chives

Instructions

SOUP

1. Boil water in a 6-quart pot. Blanch the tomatoes by placing them in boiling water for 3-5 seconds.

2. With a slotted spoon, remove the tomatoes and place them in ice water to cool for 30 seconds. Then peel the skins and remove the seeds.

3. Place the tomatoes, sherry vinegar, olive oil, and lemon juice in a blender and blend until a smooth consistency. Salt and pepper to taste.

SUCCOTASH

1. Slice onions.

2. Peel and slice garlic cloves.

3. Heat the olive oil on medium heat in a frying pan. Add onions and sauté for 2-3 minutes.

4. Add garlic cloves to the onions. Heat for another 1 minute.

5. Add green peas, fava beans, and corn kernels to the frying pan and mix together with the garlic and onions. Heat for 2-3 minutes or until soft.

6. Add lemon juice and mix.

To serve, pour the soup into bowls and place the succotash mixture in the center. Decorate with chive flowers or chives.

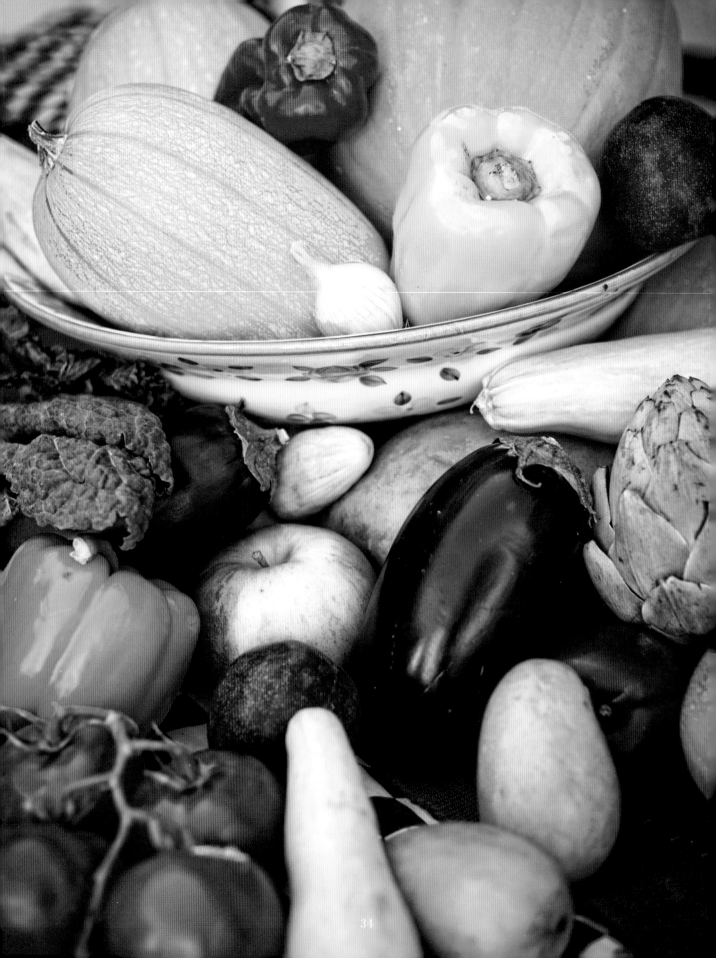

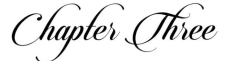

Chapter Three

Kitchen Harmonizing: Creating a Healthy Workplace

IN THE DAYS that followed I thought back on how things turned around in that Pula cave. Over time, I developed and refined a kitchen harmonizing practice that I found to really make a difference wherever I was working.

Explaining it to the Hollywood actress with the chaotic kitchen, she readily agreed to my harmonizing her space. Just like back in Pula, it made all the difference. After I harmonized, people were hanging out in her kitchen where before they never did. I was able to concentrate and work efficiently too. My client even signed a major recording contract shortly afterward. I can't prove that harmonizing her kitchen contributed to that success, of course, but my gut feeling is that I gave her a real boost. That was certainly my intention.

Word started to get around. On another occasion, a major Hollywood dealmaker hired me to harmonize his kitchen. It had everything a cook could ever need, but it was just not inviting. After I went through my harmonizing practice, the atmosphere changed. The impact was so powerful that his wife started to cook, which she had never done before. You can imagine how happy he was about that.

This idea of bringing or restoring harmony to places may be new to some people, but it's an old practice in many parts of the world. For example, feng shui has become well-known in the West, the ancient Chinese philosophy of bringing oneself and one's space into alignment with the surrounding environment. Some people even believe in building and internally arranging their homes in ways that they feel are "in sync" with the world around them. Much of the architecture in Singapore is influenced by feng shui, to which some attribute its widely acknowledged peaceful spirit.

You may not have the luxury of deciding where and how you want your kitchen to be built, but you can work with what you have to make it a place of peace and nourishment. Whether you're moving into a new home, or have simply done a lot of living in your existing home, harmonizing your kitchen can provide a fresh canvas on which you can create.

No doubt there is more than one way to harmonize a kitchen. The important thing is being aware of the energy in the room and how it can affect the food you prepare, then taking some steps to clear, purify, and balance the energy in your cooking environment.

...harmonizing your kitchen can provide a fresh canvas on which you can create.

It does not have to be complicated. These are the seven steps I follow to harmonize a kitchen.

Get Clear

The first thing is to have a clear vision for what you want in and from your kitchen. If you don't know what you are aiming for, you won't know when you have arrived, right? So what do you want for your kitchen? How do you want it to feel when you are there? What kind of effect do you want it to have on other people when they are there?

Sit in a quiet place where you can write down what comes to mind. You may come up with a clear description of what you have in mind, or simply a series of words, like **welcoming, warm, comforting, creative,** or **nourishing.**

Although I think it is important to do this without interruptions, that doesn't mean not having input from others. If you have a partner or a family, you may want to hear from them about their thoughts on this shared space.

Get Clean

Making a fresh start requires a thorough cleaning out and cleaning up. Get rid of everything you don't need. Being in a cluttered space can make you feel cluttered inside. Take time to look around at what you have and decide whether you need it.

Does your kitchen currently have an odds-and-ends drawer? Most do. It's the place where everyone puts all the things they don't know what else to do with—spare keys, tubes of superglue, foreign currency from that overseas trip you made, business cards, and many other random items.

Decide to deal with it. Go through everything there and find the right place for it, create the right place for it, or decide the right place for it is in the trash!

Imagine you will run a race, but you arrive at the start line with a bag of things you don't need strapped to your back. That will slow you down a lot. Get rid of it and you will run much more quickly. Or think about going out for a hike. If you have mud on your boots when you get home, you will bring it inside unless you take them off or clean them well.

It's the same thing in the kitchen. Not only will eliminating the junk help you feel more focused, you will discover that it's easier to find the things you do need while you cook. This will make being there more restful and fulfilling, creating an upward circle of good energy.

Organizing expert Marie Kondo has written about how your living space affects your body in her New York Times best-selling book, *The Life-Changing Magic of Tidying Up.* The Japanese author who helps clients get rid of things they don't need, to create a less cluttered home, observes that "when we reduce what we own and essentially 'detox' our house, it has a detox effect on our bodies as well."

...find the right place for it, create the right place for it,

or decide the right place for it is in the trash!

Part of the reason, she says, is because when we have less things there's less dust and it's easier for people to see what needs cleaning. In turn, with fewer things to have to worry about, she says, people also find more time to exercise and eat less junk food. "But I think the main reason tidying has this effect is because through this process people come to know contentment."

When it comes to the kitchen, Kondo recommends keeping things stored away when they are not being used. "A counter is for preparing food, not storing things," she says, pointing out that the counter space near the stove gets spattered with food and oil, making seasonings kept here "usually sticky with grease." Items kept out on the counter make it harder to clean the kitchen well.

Don't limit your cleaning to the things in your kitchen. Do the same with your food. Go through your fridge and pantry. Are there items past their sell-by date? Leftovers you haven't gotten around to doing anything with? Throw them out. You're creating physical and emotional space for more nourishing items.

As part of this cleaning, also be sure to clean up. Make a point of going over the areas you might typically overlook, like the parts of counters behind kitchen equipment, drawers, shelves, windows, and so on. In my experience, the most commonly neglected areas of the kitchen are the inside of the oven and the fridge, and the top of the fridge.

Do be sure to use biodegradable products in this whole process. Otherwise you're going to get rid of old dirt and replace it with a fresh layer of toxicity.

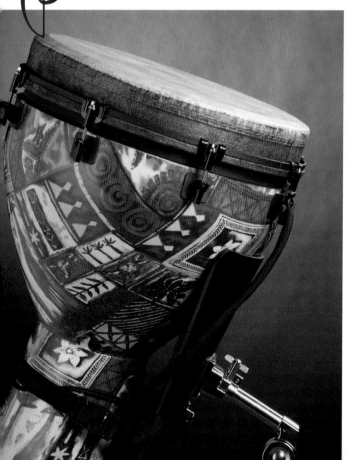

Alter the Vibration

This whole harmonizing process is intended to shake things up in your kitchen, in a good way, and now you get to do that literally. Finish your cleaning by clearing out the energy cobwebs, as it were.

I like to use my drum to shake up the energy. If you don't have one, you can also clap your hands loudly. Sustain your drumming, or clapping, for a good five minutes at least, and pay attention to the corners of the kitchen.

This may sound a little "out there" to

some people who are not used to relating to energy on a physical level, but vibrations have an impact that we cannot always see. Sound waves are one example. Or think about what happens if you clap loudly near a spider's web. You will see it vibrate and move. It is the same principle with kitchen harmonizing.

Many native cultures use drums in their rituals, because they know the rhythms have a physical impact on the environment. All physical matter vibrates, at different frequencies; we want to be sure the place where we prepare food for others "hums" well.

Preserve the Purification

Having cleaned thoroughly and drummed to "reset" the wavelength of the kitchen, I like to preserve the purifying effect. I do this in two ways. First, I take some salt and sprinkle it lightly in the corners of the room. Some different religious traditions incorporate the use of salt in rituals like house blessings. Salt is well-known for its preservative properties. It also has healing uses—some people find bathing in Epsom salts eases pain and reduces inflammation.

All physical matter vibrates, at different frequencies; we want to be sure the place where we prepare food for others "hums" well.

Second, I will ring a bell. I use one I brought back from a trip to Bali. There are many different kinds of bells out there. Find one with a tone that feels good to you, then ring away. While drumming has a hard aspect to it, shaking things up, ringing a bell is different. From schools to boxing rings, it's used to mark the end of one period of time and the start of another. Ring one to signal a new season for your kitchen.

Light Up

Candles can purify and stimulate your kitchen on an ongoing basis. I suggest you always have candles in your kitchen when you cook. Fire has long been a symbol of energy and passion, two things you want to bring to your food preparation.

Combined with color, flame can be even more powerful. Plain white candles have a meditative quality to them—not something I'd recommend when you are cooking. But consider the way these different colors can enhance and enrich the atmosphere:

- *Blue* for peacefulness.

- *Yellow* for loving energy.

- *Red* for passion and physical activity.

Baroque and Roll

We all know how music can affect our mood and performance. I'll talk more about this later, but for now think about how athletes listen to favorite tunes to pump themselves up before they compete. Lovers play romantic songs to enhance their intimacy. Worshipers turn to music to help them connect with the divine or express themselves. Filmmakers know that the right mood music can heighten the impact of a scene, from fear to great joy.

In the same way, music can set the tone for an elevated cooking experience in your newly harmonized kitchen. Baroque music—especially Bach's organ pieces—is a personal favorite of mine. When I play it as I prepare a meal, people say they can taste heaven in my food.

Experiment for yourself. Explore different kinds of music, taking time to find what resonates

---

...allow the music to flow through you

into the food you prepare.

---

best with you. Then play your favorite music and allow the music to flow through you into the food you prepare.

When you are functioning at your peak, you are in the zone. Everything you touch will be at its best. As the music releases endorphins in your body it starts a reaction that will pass through you, through your hands, and into the food you touch. You will intensify the flavor and the nourishment you offer others through your "handprint."

Plant Beauty

Finally, you should beautify your kitchen, so the environment fosters and encourages your love for others and your creativity. Introduce some cut flowers or green plants. These bring a sense of natural aliveness and freshness to the kitchen.

You can further accent the kitchen with nice art, or maybe an attractive window treatment. Make sure these are splashes of color and creativity that enhance the environment without becoming too distracting. You want them to add to the atmosphere you have created, not change it.

Treat my harmonizing outline like you would any recipe you may like. You will want to keep the main ingredients, but when you get a feel for what you're doing, you may want to modify it according to your personal preferences, adding your own special zest. But these simple steps have helped me transform some extremely unappetizing cooking environments into what have become truly sacred spaces.

Make your kitchen your own sacred space too. Happy harmonizing!

THE KELLY FAMILY'S
MEDITERRANEAN LUNCH SALAD

I made this lunch for the first time in a cave during a concert stop in Pula, Croatia. I used whatever local ingredients I could find. It quickly became a favorite of the band members who requested it repeatedly for lunch and on the weekends.

(Serves 4)

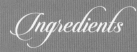

SALAD

1 16-oz. Can Garbanzo Beans

1 Tablespoon Coconut Oil

1 Golden Beet

1 Red Beet

1 Tablespoon Olive Oil

1 Cup Water

½ Cup Whole Wheat Quinoa

¼ Teaspoon Salt

¼ Teaspoon Black Pepper and Red Pepper Flakes to taste

1 Medium Size Carrot (grated)

1 Tablespoon Fresh Parsley

DRESSING

1 Tablespoon Dijon Mustard

1/8 Cup Champagne Vinegar

1 Tablespoon Raw Honey

1/8 Teaspoon Salt

¼ Teaspoon Black Pepper

¼ Cup Olive Oil

Instructions

SALAD

1. Preheat oven to 400° F.

2. Rinse and dry the garbanzo beans well. Spread them on a baking sheet and mix in 1 tablespoon coconut oil. Bake for 15-20 minutes until crunchy.

3. While the beans are cooking, cut the tops from the golden beets and red beets (cut in half if they are large).

4. Wrap all the red beets in aluminum foil and then wrap all the golden beets in aluminum foil. After removing the garbanzo beans from the oven, increase heat to 425° F. Set the garbanzo beans aside to cool.

5. Place the two bundles of red and golden beets in the oven and roast for 40-45 minutes until al dente; tender, but not mushy.

6. While the beets are roasting, boil the quinoa in 1 cup of water with 1 tablespoon of olive oil; add black peppers and red pepper flakes to taste. Simmer until water evaporates and the quinoa is soft.

7. Remove beets from the oven and let cool. When cool enough to handle, remove the skin and grate them. Set aside.

8. Grate the carrot and put aside.

9. Chop 1 tablespoon fresh parsley.

10. Make the dressing.

DRESSING

1. In a blender, mix all the ingredients (except the olive oil) until smooth. Slowly add the olive oil to emulsify.

2. To serve: On a large plate, arrange the garbanzo beans in a circular pattern on the outside of the plate. Then, working inward, add the beets and carrots. Place the quinoa in the middle.

3. Gently pour the dressing over the salad items on the plate and decorate with chopped parsley.

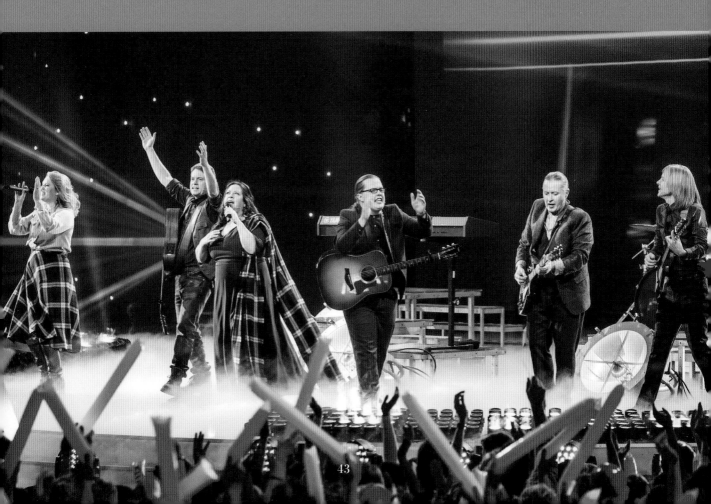

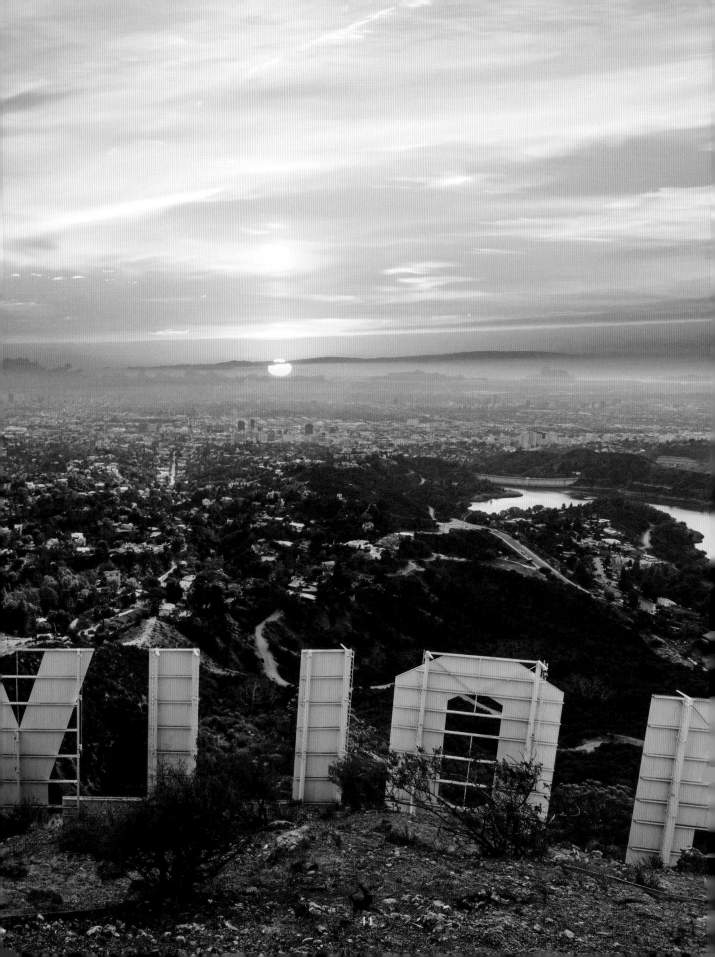

Chapter Four

A Taste of Celebrity Life Behind the Scenes

THE FIRST TIME we met, Bob Hope kissed me twice and said, "Don't tell my wife!"

I had found my way to his Toluca Lake-area home with the directions from Chris, my new agent in Los Angeles, but at first I thought I must have gone to the wrong door. It was opened by Dennis, the Hopes' personal manager, who invited me in. I stepped into the kitchen, and there sitting at a table was the legendary comedian and actor himself.

He greeted me, and then looked curious when I replied.

"Where are you from?" he asked, having noted my Hebrew accent overshadowing the English words I spoke.

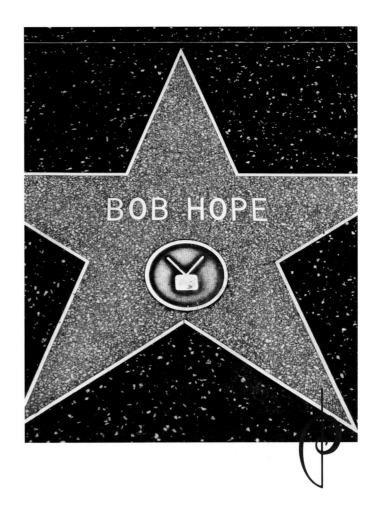

When I told him I was from Israel, he beamed. Jumping up from the table, he came over and kissed me on both cheeks in affection. Having jokingly told me not to tell his wife, Dolores, he clapped his hands in delight.

"I love Israel," he declared. "When your country was just born, I came and sang for your soldiers. I fell in love with your country and your people. I support Israel every year."

As we were speaking, Dolores came into the room and Bob told her about my background.

She smiled and then asked me a few questions.

Almost before I knew it, they said, "We want to hire you." They told Dennis to work out the details for my contract, which would be for several months while their usual chef was unavailable because of a family situation.

I didn't know much about the celebrity chef world, but I did realize this swift process was rather unorthodox. There's usually a longer interview and some sort of demonstration of your cooking skills required.

When Dennis asked me what my fee was I was caught flat-footed. I did not know I should have referred him to Chris for these details, so I plucked a figure out of the air. I knew it was pretty high, but Dennis made clear quite how much.

"That's more than the permanent chef makes," he said. "But they really seemed to like you, so I'm going to go and ask them. Wait here."

Five minutes later he was back.

"You've got the position," he told me.

Determined to make a good impression, I decided to beautify Dolores's first breakfast tray. I went out into the garden, where there was an incredible array of rose bushes for which the Hopes were famous. Dolores loved roses, retaining a gardener to care for the hundreds they grew on the property and hosting tours of their collection to raise money for charity.

Some of the Hopes' other staff were horrified when they learned that I had clipped one of Dolores's beloved flowers. They warned me not to set it on her tray, but I felt it gave the setting a little flourish so I went ahead anyway.

Dolores never said a word about the "transgression" when I brought in her food. So every day after that I would clip a fresh rose to decorate the tray. Only one time did she comment, telling me I could cut from any of the bushes except the one bearing a rare black flower. I made sure to steer clear of that one.

A Little Chutzpah

Leaving that first celebrity position with the Hope family at the end of my contract with a glowing letter of recommendation, I had also learned a lot about how to work with and for wealthy and famous clients.

One lesson was the importance of a certain amount of chutzpah, the Yiddish way of describing a little bit of cheekiness or audacity. I was always respectful of my clients, but I was not intimidated by them. My attitude was that I was there to serve them, but I was not their servant. I expected them to treat me courteously as I did them. For the most part that was my experience.

This refusal to be overawed by people of stature goes way back to my childhood. I was around four years of age when Yoram came to collect me from kindergarten class one day and we noticed all sorts of activity outside a house we walked by every day on the way home. There were many vehicles parked alongside the road and people standing all around.

I asked Yoram what was going on. He said that David Ben-Gurion, Israel's beloved first Prime Minister, had come from Jerusalem to visit the friends of ours who lived there.

"I want to see him!" I said. "I want to see him!"

Yoram took me to the front door and we knocked. We were greeted by the woman of the house who asked what we wanted.

"My sister wants to see David Ben-Gurion," Yoram told her.

"All right," she said, surprising us both. "Do you want to see him too?"

Yoram said no, that he would wait outside. The woman took me by the hand and walked me into a rear room where Ben-Gurion was sitting with his wife and several other people. I don't know whether it was some sort of a government meeting, or just an informal gathering.

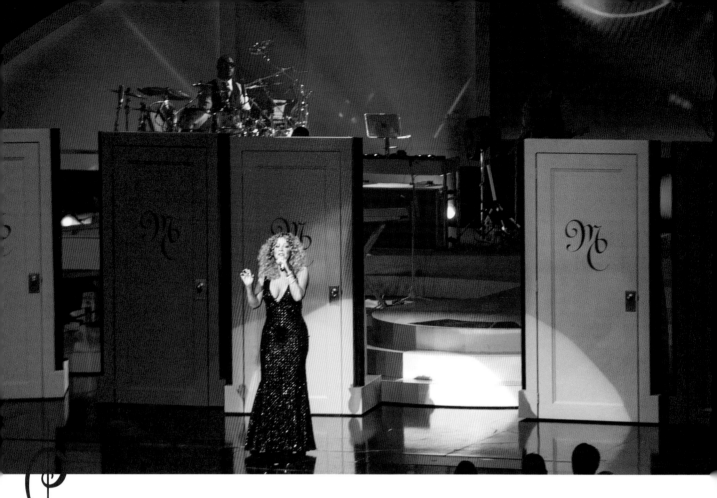

After I had been introduced, Paula Ben-Gurion looked at my skinny frame and said, "I see that you don't like to eat." Then she sat me on her husband's lap and proceeded to feed me pita bread dipped in hummus and eggplant salad.

My visit lasted only a few minutes, but something about being welcomed and accepted even though I might have been considered an interruption must have stuck with me. I have never since been nervous in the presence of famous people.

That chutzpah was how I came to spoon-feed Mariah Carey during my interview and end up touring the world with her—even teaching her to dance to the traditional Israeli folk song "Hava Nagila" along the way.

Over the Rainbow

I got a call from my agent, Chris, telling me Mariah's people were looking for a private chef to join the singer on her world tour in 2000 in support of her latest album release,

Rainbow, which was to begin soon.

I was one of several candidates being considered, and spoke about my background and experience in the interview. At some point, something just welled up inside me and I said, "All I want is to take care of Mariah." That spontaneous comment must have struck a chord, because the next thing I knew, I had been given the job.

Before finalizing things, I had to meet Mariah, naturally. I waited quite some time, as she was busy finalizing some video work, but eventually she came to say hello. I was familiar with her music, and knew that she was a true superstar. But I immediately found her to be very friendly and warm.

We chatted pleasantly for a while, and she told me she would like to sample some of my food before making a final decision. "I love everything," she told me, "except curry powder. Don't give me curry."

"Right," I replied. "Madame Carey does not like curry!"

She laughed.

The next day I returned with a fresh serving of my famous roasted red and yellow pepper soup, something I thought would be the right balance of flavorful and nutritious.

With the tour starting soon, Mariah was caught up in a flurry of last-minute preparations. I was ushered in to where she was working, but she was distracted by all the demands being made of her.

If it gets too cold it just isn't going to taste the same, I thought. She needs to try it while it is still warm.

Drawing close with the bowl, I dipped the spoon into it and held it to Mariah's lips as she looked at a computer screen. She took a sip, then another.

"It tastes sweet," she said, turning to me with a smile. "Just like you." I was hired.

In my *Rainbow* tour travels I got to see Mariah close up. Though she exuded confidence and charisma on stage, away from the lights she could be quiet, almost shy. Partly she had to conserve her energy for the next show. There would be days when she needed to rest her voice and would communicate only by writing notes.

With around one hundred and fifty people as part of the Rainbow tour crew, two big trucks were needed each time we landed to transport all the luggage to the hotel. My main job was to provide lunch and dinner—something light enough not to leave her feeling heavy and tired but with enough nutrition to sustain her through a demanding performance—and some simple snacks for the green room. Mariah ate a lot of vegetables, with salmon and saltwater fish as her favorites, along with my signature frittatas.

I would be given the run of the kitchens of the five-star hotels in which we stayed, with a chauffeur to take me out to buy whatever ingredients I wanted and a "spend what you need to" credit card. Then I would serve Mariah in her private suite. Often she would ask me to sit with her as she ate, and she would tell me about her life, and growing up.

After the Applause

Though concerts and appearances are physically draining, they also leave performers on an adrenaline high afterward, when it can be hard to come down. I'd often serve herbal teas to help soothe wired nerves. Chamomile was especially calming, I found.

Entertainers will often be very hungry after finishing a show and giving of themselves so physically, but I learned they needed something light, not heavy like pasta. After I had served The Kelly Family post-show, I would make sure that only quiet, relaxing music was playing in the background, to help bring them down, rather than sounds that kept them amped up.

One night on the *Rainbow* tour after one of the concerts, my room phone rang. It was Mariah.

"Honey," she said, "I cannot go to sleep. Could you please make me one of your special egg dishes?"

Dressing quickly, I went down to the kitchen and got busy with the eggs and made one of my famous frittatas, which I knew Mariah enjoyed. When I arrived with the food she wanted some company. I enjoyed my time with her, and we sat for an hour or so chatting.

As with all my other clients, I felt that I was not just feeding Mariah's body but feeding her soul too. I wanted her to feel good about herself and the world, believing that when she was feeling at her best she could offer her best.

The way good food prepared with love and care can bring joy and togetherness was sweetly illustrated for me when the *Rainbow* tour reached Italy.

We were staying at Milan's renowned Four Seasons Hotel when Mariah decided she wanted to cook her personal staff a special meal. That inner-circle group included her manager, her stylists, video editor, and me.

Mariah chose her specialty—pasta with clams. As her "sous chef" I enjoyed cooking with her and helping with the preparations. Then she diligently finished things off and served all of us. The intimate gathering put us all in a fun, silly mood. At one point, I asked Mariah why, if she was from Queens, she did not speak with any hint of a New York accent?

"You want New York?" She chuckled and launched into a lengthy monologue in the city's most striking tones.

Then she turned to me.

"Z," she said, using the affectionate nickname she gave me, "you're from Israel. Can you sing something in Hebrew? I'd really like to hear it."

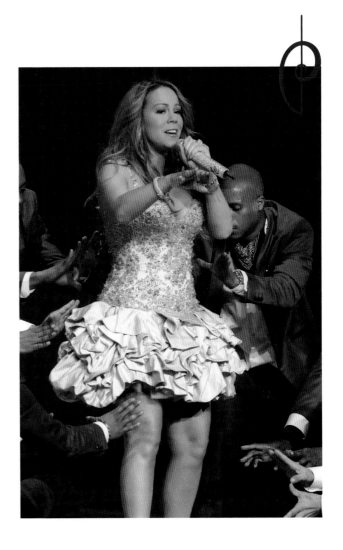

Without stopping to think that I was singing in front of someone with one of the most wonderful voices in the world, I opened my mouth and started to sing:

Hava nagila

Hava nagila

Hava nagila ve-nismeha

I stood up to demonstrate the familiar, joyous steps that go with the song. Mariah and the others stood to join in, and soon we were all dancing and laughing. Then my voice cracked between notes, and we all laughed some more.

As I got to know her better, I took on responsibility for meeting more of Mariah's personal needs. When we arrived at a new hotel, I would make sure the pillows in her room were of the right thread count, her favorite wine was chilling in the fridge, the flowers just so, and the humidifiers were running properly to protect her voice.

Such attention to detail may make celebrities sound high maintenance, and some can be very particular. But remember that as the center of a major business operation they have a very stressful position, so I have always felt anything I can do to help ease that is not only caring for them personally but in some way for all the other people who are part of their world.

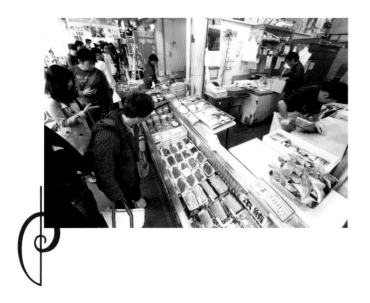

Being part of a world-famous artist's inner circle opened the door to all kinds of experiences. On Mariah's *Rainbow* tour I was able to fulfill a long-held dream of visiting Tokyo's renowned Tsukiji fish market. The largest fish and seafood market in the world, famed especially for its tuna, with its nearly one thousand stalls it's almost like a small city, vibrating with activity, humming with noise, and swirling with smells.

My driver took me there before sunrise, to see Tsukiji at its busiest. There seemed to be every variety of fish possible there—and some I did not even recognize. It was fascinating to see the fresh catches of tuna being auctioned.

Among the market's attractions is a celebrated sushi bar. It doesn't look much to the casual passerby—small, with room for maybe only a dozen or so people. You don't get to choose, you just eat what you are presented with. But people wait for up to two hours to be served. It's worth every moment, I can testify.

I've enjoyed some good sushi in the United States in my time, and consider myself a bit of a connoisseur, but I have never tasted any like that I enjoyed at Tsukiji. Just one of the perks of life as a celebrity chef.

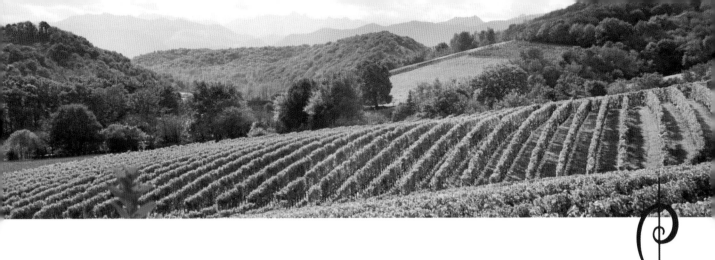

Keeping the Stars Shining

Over time, I almost became part of the family with some of my clients. That was never more true than with The Kelly Family, with whom I lived and traveled more than any other client.

Our time together included three months at famed Chateau Miraval in the south of France, an estate with its own recording studio and vineyard later owned by Brad Pitt and Angelina Jolie. We stayed there while the band recorded an album in the studio, also used by the likes of the Gypsy Kings, Pink Floyd, Sade, and Sting. I especially enjoyed preparing meals featuring some of the many delicious cheeses from the region, and matching them with wine from the chateau's own grounds.

Spending so much time together in one place, away from the busy schedule of the road, we grew even closer, and the Kellys all became very dear to me. Our fond relationship was broadcast live in Germany one time when we appeared on a daytime television show. Loved all over Europe, where they would often be mobbed when out in public, the Kellys were superstars in Germany, and we had been asked into the studio for a segment about how they lived and ate on the road.

I was supposed to demonstrate how I prepared their favorite fresh Irish soda bread, a delicious whole wheat brown loaf. All was going well until one of the siblings, Maite, playfully tossed flour in my face. Without thinking, I threw some back at her, and then there we all were, having a fun food fight on German television.

Being able to read just what my clients needed from me to succeed in eating healthily was important. They differed in the way they received motivation. For some it was the friendly encouragement of a friend or older sister. For others I needed to be more of their Jewish momma or a firm schoolteacher.

Learning the dietary requirements of the different artists I worked with was a bit like being a tailor, trimming the fabrics to fit their unique person.

One time I caught a client, who was on a strict eating program to hit a deadline for getting in shape, with a donut in their hand. Then I found contraband pudding in the fridge. I scolded them in a good-natured way, but made it clear that I was there to help them succeed. I also threatened to increase my fee if they didn't keep on track. I don't know whether it was the telling off or the fear of being "fined," but they accepted my tough love message.

Learning the dietary requirements of the different artists I worked with was a bit like being a tailor, trimming the fabrics to fit their unique person. I'd consult with their doctor and nutritionist if they had a strict health or fitness regime they were following. From there it was a mix of science and art, avoiding foods before a performance that might leave the client feeling parched, or bloated, or gassy. That ruled out spicy foods, which constrict the throat, or things like tomatoes or oranges, which are known for pinching the vocal chords.

Some preferred to stick to tried-and-true menus, while others liked to be more adventurous. Seal was working on a new CD in the state-of-the-art personal recording studio he had in his Hollywood home when I was contracted to provide lunch and dinner daily for him and his crew, for a season. He wanted something different every meal, which stretched my creativity.

I served everything from Indian to Mediterranean cuisine. He must have been happy with what I came up with, because he then asked me to cater a weekly, Friday night dinner at which he hosted some of the music industry's leading figures. One time I decided to prepare about twenty-five small lobsters, and he offered to help. He told me stories about his childhood as we sat together in the kitchen cracking the shells.

The kitchen adjoined the studio, which led to an amusing incident. In the afternoons, Seal would be visited by a man and I'd hear the strangest noises coming through the wall. It sounded for all the world like someone was trying to kill a cow, or some kind of tribal ritual.

One afternoon, the visitor came into the kitchen for some reason, and we chatted a little. My curiosity got the better of me, and I knew I had to take the opportunity to find out.

"What was all the noise about?" I asked. "Was it some kind of incantation or ancient credo?"

"Oh no." The man laughed. "I'm a vocal coach. That's one of the exercises we do."

For all his openness to variety, there was one thing about which Seal was very definite—his afternoon tea. He knew just how he wanted his "cuppa" to be prepared. On my first day working with him he explained about boiling the water and how long to let the tea leaves steep before pouring.

One day I got distracted and left the tea leaves in too long. But there was no time to throw it away and make a fresh cup, so I decided to serve it up and hope for the best. A little later he came and told me that had been the best cup I'd ever made. So much for routine.

While I thoroughly enjoyed working with celebrity clients, over time I found the constant demands beginning to wear on me. I was so focused on caring for them and making sure they were doing well that I was not looking after myself enough. Long days ensuring they were eating healthily and looking and feeling good left me tired. Gradually my weight increased, until one day I realized I was now a size sixteen.

I was horrified. I recognized that I wasn't living what I was "preaching" to others. Some people think the round, jolly chef is the ultimate advertisement for their food, but not me. I knew I needed to live more consistently with what I believed and encouraged in others.

About the same time, I was asked whether I would like to be the private chef for singer Mick Jagger. It was a great opportunity, and I knew the Rolling Stones frontman seriously cared for his health and weight, and would be someone great to work with. But I also knew I needed to take some time out to focus on myself.

Leaving Los Angeles, I moved to Scottsdale, Arizona, to regroup. With the support and encouragement of good friends, I spent time taking better care of myself and studying more about dietary health. Refreshed and refocused, I developed a more comprehensive philosophy and approach to food and health that could be attainable by anyone, even if they didn't have a private chef.

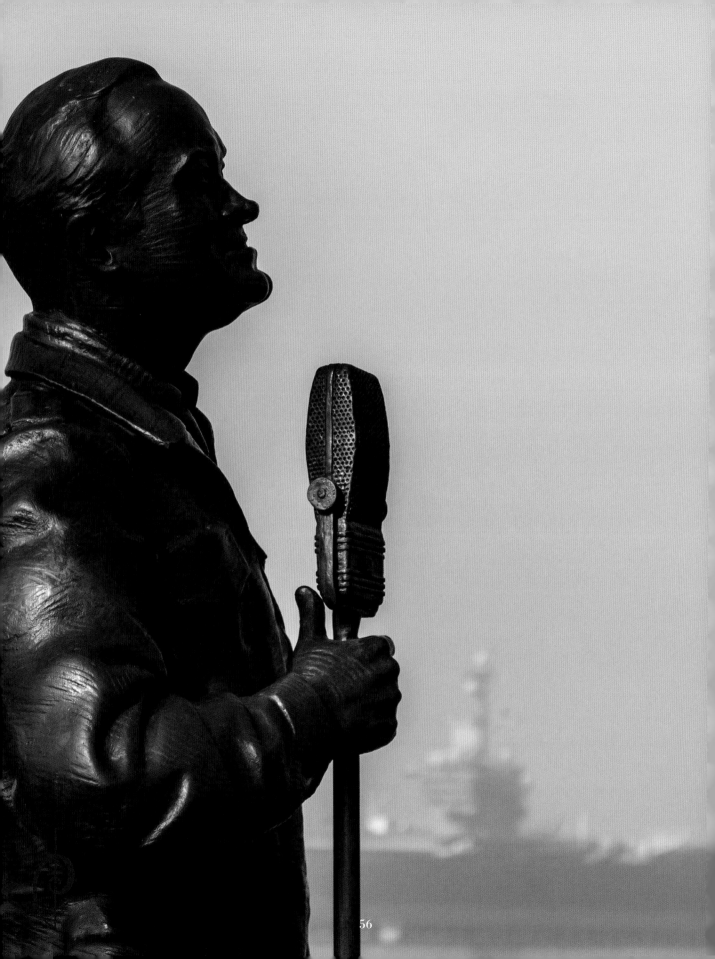

BOB AND DOLORES HOPE'S PROSCIUTTO ROASTED FRESH FIGS

The Hopes' gardens were most famous for Dolores's beautiful roses, but their grounds also contained two wonderful fig trees; one purple, one green. They asked me to cook a dish using the fresh figs (you can substitute apricots when figs are not in season). I created two special appetizers.

PROSCIUTTO ROASTED FRESH FIGS

(Appetizer Serves 15-20)

Ingredients

40 Fresh Figs
(available in season only)

4 oz. Blue Cheese

4 oz. Thin-sliced Prosciutto

Salt and Pepper to taste

Instructions

1. Preheat oven to 400° F.
2. Slice each fig; make a pocket and fill it with blue cheese, then wrap with the prosciutto.
3. Bake 12-15 minutes.
4. Serve on a platter.

ROASTED FIGS APPETIZER

(Appetizer Serves 4)

Ingredients

12 Fresh Figs

1-2 Tablespoons Powdered Sugar

2 Tablespoons Balsamic Vinegar (good quality, aged)

2 Tablespoons Water

5 Tablespoons Sugar

1 Packet Non-Salty Butter

Instructions

1. Preheat oven to 375° F.
2. Slice figs in half.
3. Combine powdered sugar and balsamic vinegar; put aside.
4. Place the white sugar in a skillet on medium heat; dissolve until caramelized to a dark amber color. Do not mix.
5. Add the butter, 1 tablespoon balsamic vinegar, and water.
6. Heat the ingredients in the skillet for 1 minute and then add figs; heat for another 3 minutes and remove from the heat.
7. Remove the figs from sauce and place in a dish lined with parchment paper.
8. Bake in oven for 5 minutes.
9. Remove and place on a platter. Sprinkle with the powdered sugar and balsamic.

Serve with fresh ricotta cheese, orange peel, and chopped unsalted pistachios.

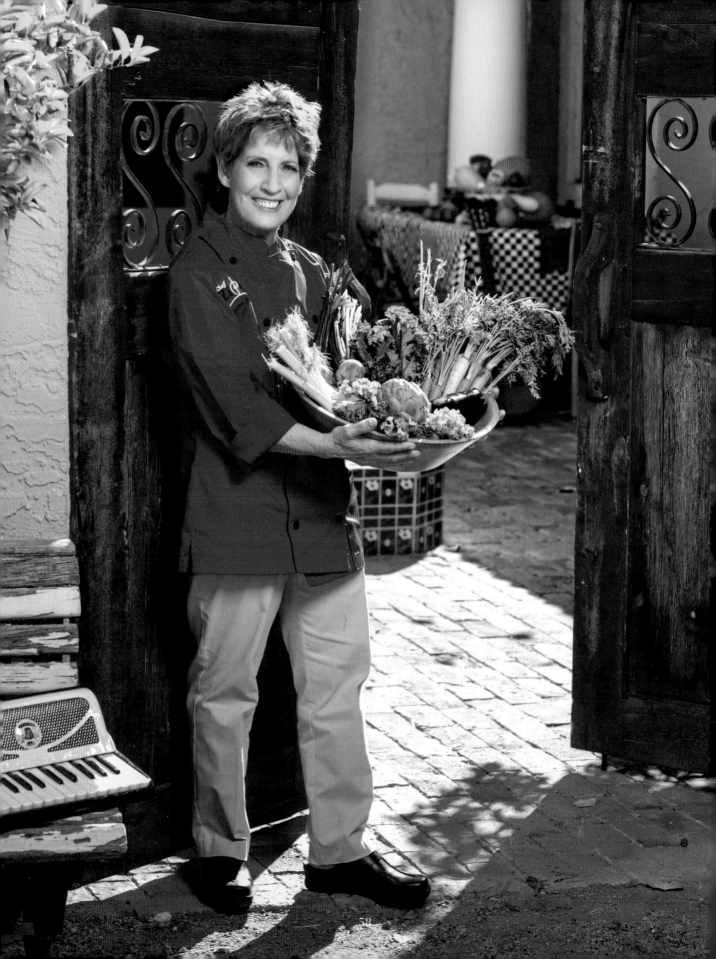

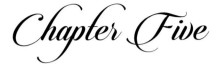

Harmonizing Your Inner World

YOU HAVE PROBABLY heard it said that there is nothing quite like a home-cooked meal. Some of my celebrity clients could have afforded the fanciest ingredients, but they were most content with simple fare they remembered from their childhood.

Perhaps there are basic things you had as a kid that you still eat with delight now? And then you might go to a fancy restaurant and have a gourmet meal, only to find that after time you get tired of eating out, even in a five-star setting. What's that about?

Chances are your mother wasn't as good a cook as some of the great ones you will find at five-star restaurants. Nor were her recipes likely to be that special. And she may not have had access to the same high-quality ingredients. But what she probably had that restaurants too often don't was a genuine feeling for the people who are consuming the food.

You might say that best intentions are more important than best abilities or best ingredients. As Mozart once remarked, "Neither a lofty degree of intelligence nor imagination nor both together go to the making of genius. Love, love, love, that is the soul of genius."

At the end of the day, it's not what's on the menu that is the most important thing, it's who's behind the kitchen door. As I have said, the environment in which food is being prepared is important, but so is the person who does it.

More than just the recipes and ingredients, the care and love with which they are prepared are what sets good food apart. That's what people are craving when they ask for childhood favorite meals; the love their mom (usually) put into what she served up. Conversely, food prepared without a lot of care and concern is simply not as satisfying—and I write as someone who knows that firsthand, from my own childhood.

No wonder our appetites often aren't satiated. After all, we're not just consuming someone's cooking, we're taking in the lack of energy and indifferent attitude with which those dishes were prepared.

I was already aware of some of this when I was traveling as private chef to The Kelly Family band. But I was fascinated to stumble across an article in a magazine, as we waited at London's Heathrow Airport for a flight to Ireland, that confirmed what I had been sensing.

I read about an experiment in which a man was placed in a comfortable room and served the same meal on three different occasions. Each time he ate, his vital signs were measured to track the physiological effects. He was also interviewed for his personal response.

With each meal, his vital signs and verbal feedback would vary somewhat. Most dramatically, after one of the meals the man's blood pressure shot up, and he reported how the food tasted bitter and he experienced feelings of hostility.

What the volunteer didn't know was that the meals had been prepared using the same ingredients—but by three different people. And the person who had prepared the meal that left him feeling sick had been a prisoner.

Learning about this experiment got me excited. It helped clarify for me why all my life people had told me they felt special when eating my food, from my brother Yoram to celebrities such as Mariah Carey and Pierce Brosnan.

It also helped me understand why, throughout my career, if ever I was in an angry mood, I never wanted to touch food. Clearly, who we are at the moment when we cook affects the people who eat it. It is like we add an invisible, emotional seasoning to the food that we prepare.

The potential power of cooking with heart was made even clearer to me when I read the book *The Hidden Messages in Water* by Masaru Emoto. In it he described experiments in which water molecules were affected by their exposure to words, pictures, and music conveying different emotions, and how when frozen the crystals formed pleasant or ugly shapes, depending on the "message" they had received.

Some have questioned the scientific validity of his research, but Emoto's foundational belief that negative or positive energy has the power to affect living things rang true to me. There's no doubt in my mind that food being prepared is even more vulnerable than water to the feelings of people around it, specifically the cook. This is because cooking is an act of creation, where raw ingredients are transformed into dishes and meals. During this transformation, the ingredients are in the hands of the cook, and I believe they take on that person's character at that moment.

Even before reading Emoto's book, I was aware our hands can be channels of healing and comfort. Think about how masseurs work the knots and kinks out of people's bodies, leaving them feeling calm and peaceful. In some religious traditions, priests will lay hands on people to pray for their healing.

For as long as I could remember, people had commented when I would hug or touch them kindly that they felt a warmth or comfort. That feedback had encouraged me to study reiki, the Japanese alternative healing technique of stress reduction and relaxation based on releasing the life force in someone through touch. I'd sometimes use it on clients I was especially close with, such as The Kelly Family, who found it helpful after an intense show.

Being reminded of the mind-body-spirit connection became part of the reason for my eventually stepping away from the celebrity world, for a while. Overweight and unhappy, I felt like I wasn't being entirely honest with my clients. I wanted them to look and feel and be their best, but inside I was struggling with self-esteem that was surely going to seep through in the food that I made.

You can have the most harmonized, tidiest kitchen, but if you are simmering in resentment or stewing in anger, you are going to contaminate the food that you prepare.

Since then I have learned that just as it's important to harmonize your kitchen, it's also very important for you to come into the kitchen to prepare food in a state of personal, inner harmony. Having cleaned the space and the equipment, we also need to clear our thoughts and attitudes, so we can be clean vessels.

Starting Out Well

You can have the most harmonized, tidiest kitchen, but if you are simmering in resentment or stewing in anger, you are going to contaminate the food that you prepare.

With this in mind, I aim to start each day by ensuring I am centered and at peace with myself and the world around me. My morning ritual takes about an hour, but I know it's important, so if that means setting the alarm very early because I have to be somewhere first thing for an appointment, I will.

Meditation helps me clear my mind. I will listen to classical music, which I find to be calming, especially Bach. Somehow relaxing and focusing on the music helps bring me to my highest, purest frequency. Ideally I'll do this for twenty minutes or so, but that's not always possible. Even five minutes is beneficial.

Then I think of the people I love and care for, and turn my thoughts to them. Though I consider myself to be spiritual, I am not a religious person, so I would not say that I pray, but I hold them in my thoughts and wish them well. I finish by spending a few moments focused on gratitude, bringing to mind a particular person or situation for which I am thankful.

You will want to develop your own daily practice, one that fits your beliefs. Forgiveness, gratitude, and being present to the world are universal principles that are accessible to everyone, whether they are atheist, Buddhist, Christian, Jewish, Muslim, or something else.

Generally speaking, I am a happy person by nature, so I don't find it difficult to be positive—though I am not saying I don't face difficulties and challenges, of course. We all do. That's part of life. But I have always made it a point not to hold on to resentments or negative feelings. Why be envious of someone else's success? Why not instead be glad for them and still desire the same good results for yourself? Why not look for the positive?

I'm reminded of the story of an experiment involving twin brothers from a wealthy family, Johnny and Bobby. Johnny was happy no matter what, while Bobby was the exact opposite.

The boys were put alone in separate rooms, where they were secretly observed. Bobby was placed in a room with just about every kind of toy you could imagine, everything a child could dream of, but it wasn't enough. He complained about everything. Why did he get this model instead of that one, and so on.

Meanwhile, Johnny was led into a room with just a pile of horse manure and a shovel. He began enthusiastically digging away, and when asked why, he answered, "Well, with all this manure, there's got to be a pony around here somewhere."

Attitude makes all the difference!

Learning to Let Go

I try to remember Johnny's example when I face a challenge. If I argue with somebody close to me, I allow myself to feel upset for a few minutes but I decide not to be angry. It's a choice. Sometimes I have to talk to myself, or sometimes I have to listen to music or go do something to help me get back on track, but at the end of the day I don't let my emotions—particularly the dark ones, which we all have—dominate.

Focusing negatively on what someone else did to me or didn't do for me doesn't help in the long run. I'm the one who loses. And then all that internal toxicity builds up in me, and I pass it on as I prepare food for others. Directly or indirectly, through our words and actions or the "contaminated" food we prepare, we give the negativity inside us to other people.

Though you may do all you can personally to keep the kitchen energy positive, you can't always account for what other people bring in. Do avoid fighting in the kitchen whenever possible, though. I suggest to my clients that they build a shed outside their house and take any fights they may have out there! Of course things come up from time to time and

---

Remember, the kitchen is the heart of your home,

so treat it with tenderness.

---

we don't always know how to resolve them right away. Disagreements happen, but don't let them drag on and on. Unresolved disputes drain the life out of you and your kitchen. Remember, the kitchen is the heart of your home, so treat it with tenderness.

The intention you put into your food preparation should reflect the feelings you have for the people for whom you are cooking. This isn't just a test of your love: you can love someone and still not feel particularly excited about cooking for them, just like my mom. But without the passion of the cook, the food is never quite as tasty, satisfying, or nourishing.

The power of food to communicate personal feeling is beautifully captured in a couple of movies I love. Like *Water for Chocolate*, based on the novel by Laura Esquivel, centers on Tita, the daughter of a Mexican family, who is barred from marriage by family tradition until her mother dies. She falls in love but the man is refused Tita's hand by her mother, who instead offers the older sister in marriage. The man accepts, but only to be near Tita.

Forbidden to be with the man she loves, Tita pours all her emotions into her cooking—with dramatic results. The cake she makes for her sister's wedding leaves all the guests sick. A year later Tita imbues a quail dish with her latent sexual desires, and her other sister is carried off naked by a soldier of the Revolution.

In the movie *Babette's Feast*, two spinster sisters are awakened to long-ignored pleasures when the refugee woman who has served as their housekeeper and cook for many years uses money she wins in a lottery to prepare a sumptuous meal for the women and their friends. They gradually come alive as they allow themselves to experience the delights set before them.

While the magical style of the movies takes the point to the extreme, it's no great stretch of the imagination to see how attitudes and emotions are captured in the food we prepare. So the question is—what do you want to feed your family and friends? Here are some tips for making sure your cooking comes straight from the heart.

- Never cook out of resentment. Ask yourself, "Do I want to cook for these people?" If the answer is yes, then do so with joy. If the answer is no, then don't cook.

- Never cook out of obligation. This is a tough one, especially for parents who've already had a hard day's work and may not have a lot of energy left to pour into preparing a meal for the family. "What am I supposed to do?" you may wonder. Everyone needs to eat.

My answer: if you're going to put the energy into cooking, you might as well do it with love in your heart. This love won't drain you further. In fact, your purpose in cooking, to nourish your family or guests as deeply as possible, will give you more energy and help make the food delicious and healthy.

Take a little time to get in touch with your core feelings for the people you're going to cook for. By this I mean your deepest emotions, those beneath the surface. That means that even if you've had a recent disagreement or fight, you're not letting that carry over into your cooking.

One way to do this is to think of the best qualities of the person. This will help you focus on what you appreciate about them, rather than what you dislike. If you can't think of anything, you probably shouldn't be cooking for them!

- Work in a beautiful environment. Flowers, candles, and music can all help elevate your mood. Put these kitchen harmonizing principles to work. You'll be impressed by the results.

- Seek feedback. Cooking is itself a form of communication, so you will want to hear back from the people for whom you are preparing food. Talk with your family and find out what they like to eat. Explain to them you want feedback, not criticism. You don't want to be put down. You want input that inspires you, that keeps you fresh and on your toes.

- Don't be afraid to ask for some appreciation. If you're taken for granted, you're going to lose your edge. Your passion will fade and cooking will become just another chore on the to-do list. I fired two clients for precisely this reason.

They paid me well, but they had no appreciation for my food. Every day they came up with new complaints. It's natural for people not to like one dish or another—everyone's tastes are unique. But these two could never get specific in their criticism. They just "didn't like" whatever I came up with. Their feedback wasn't in any way constructive.

I realized they were two wealthy but very unhappy people who didn't feel good about themselves and therefore didn't feel good about anyone else. Every time I saw their name on my phone's caller ID, I didn't want to answer. Their negativity was like secondhand smoking. It was affecting everyone around them, and I didn't want that.

"We hope you don't take it personally," they said to me. "This is just our personality."

"Of course I take it personally," I said as kindly as I could. "You're negating all my energy—even for other people. It's not fair to me or to my other clients." I told them that I was sorry, but I could only cook for people who liked my food, otherwise I couldn't put my full intention into my work.

Intention works both way. The eater has to reciprocate. This creates an endless cycle of

Intention produces a frequency that is as real as any radio signal...

giving and receiving. One feeds into the other (no pun intended)—the cook nourishes the eaters, and the eaters in turn nourish the cook. You're inspired, and your food preparation becomes more and more elevated. Intention produces a frequency that is as real as any radio signal, one that impacts the food for the better or for the worse. It's not something you learn so much as something you live.

Although I have gotten unusually positive reactions to my cooking all my life, I have never taken it for granted. In the early days, I used to be shocked when I got generous compliments, particularly because I never had any formal training. Self-taught, learning from books and from watching TV, but mostly from simple trial-and-error cooking, I didn't always know what I was doing, but I always put my heart into it. Yet people seemed to taste the positive intention.

They would tell me, "When I eat your food, I feel positive," or "I feel like I want to exercise," and "I feel like I want to go make a sale!" When Mariah Carey told me my pepper soup was "sweet like me," she may not have meant it literally. But my intention truly was to nourish her and apparently this came across.

THE KELLY FAMILY'S IRISH SODA BREAD

Heralding from Cove, Ireland, a tiny one-pub village near Cork, the Kelly's loved their familiar Irish soda bread. It was a taste of home for them, so I cooked several loaves each day!

Ingredients

2 Cups Whole-Wheat Flour

2 Cups Unbleached All-Purpose Flour

1-2/3 Teaspoons Sea Salt

1 Teaspoon Baking Soda

2 Cups Low-Fat Buttermilk

3 Tablespoons Honey

Instructions

1. Preheat oven to 400° F.

2. Spray a 9-inch x 5-inch bread loaf pan with olive oil spray. Line with parchment paper and spray with more olive oil.

3. In a medium bowl, mix the dry ingredients (whole-wheat flour, all-purpose flour, sea salt, and baking soda).

4. In a small bowl, mix together well the buttermilk and honey.

5. Using a spoon, make a hole in the middle of the dry ingredients mixture. Pour in the buttermilk and honey mixture and gently stir together using a fork.

6. On the counter, spread fresh flour on the counter and gently knead the dough.

7. Place the dough in the bread loaf pan.

8. Lower the oven to 375° F.

9. Bake 50-60 minutes to a deep golden brown, until toothpick tests clean.

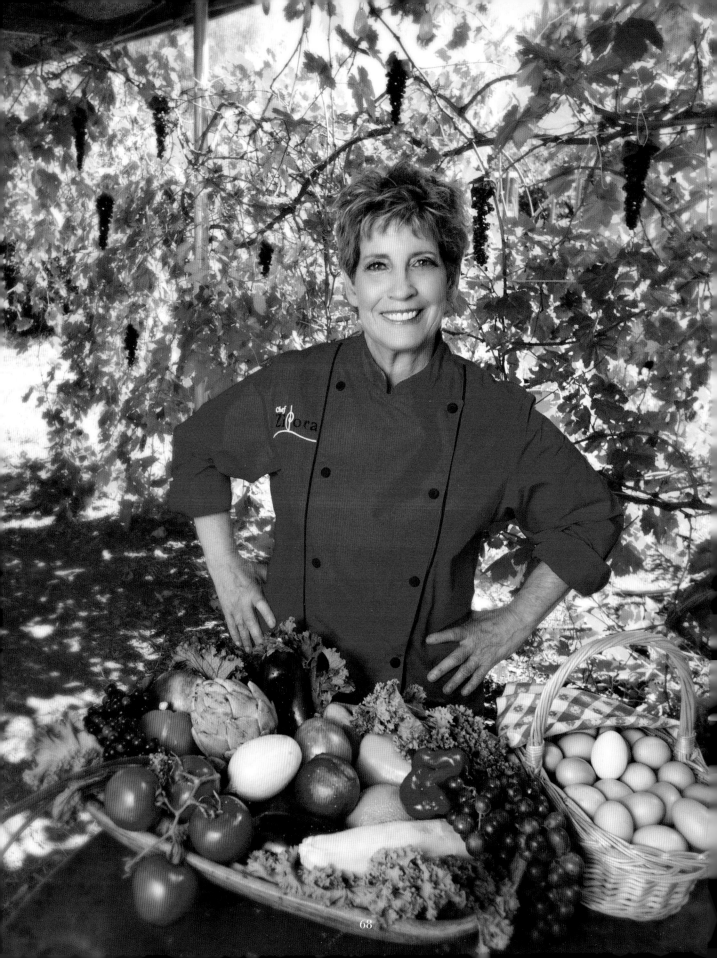

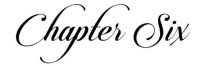

How to Embrace Change

LOOKING GOOD AND being fit may not seem to be quite as essential for your life as for the music, movie, and sports stars I have worked with. After all, no one is going to mind if you're carrying a few extra pounds when you get to your desk at the office, or if you are at home with children.

But feeling good about yourself is important whatever you are doing. If you are healthy and happy you have more life to enjoy and share with others. And who doesn't want that? The lessons I have learned working with celebrity clients are applicable to everyone, regardless of their status.

If you want to address your weight and well-being, the first thing I want to tell you is: be gentle to yourself! If charity begins at home, as the saying goes, then loving others well needs to start with loving yourself well. We can only pass on to others what we have ourselves. I like the way Bridgette Becker, a therapeutic certified nutrition consultant and holistic health practitioner, puts it: "Love yourself enough to let your food choices be an act of self-care."

Be assured you can get to the weight you want to be. You can gain the energy you need. And you can look and feel great while doing it. You can have your cake and eat it too. Well, okay, maybe not your cake necessarily, but some other delicious dishes!

You can have it all—a great shape without going hungry or making yourself sick. In fact, you can feel stronger and more alive than you ever have.

Perhaps like many clients who have come to me wanting to change their eating habits, you know just about everything there is to know about carbs, proteins, sugars, and fats.

...you can feel stronger and more alive than you ever have.

However, like them you continue to struggle with your weight, energy, and inspiration. What's going on here? You are weighed down—not just by your food choices, but by your history with food. In the words of the well-known song from Disney's *Frozen* movie, you've got to "Let It Go"!

If you have not succeeded in making the breakthrough changes you want with your weight and well-being in the past, I want to tell you: failure is not the end, it is just the beginning. But you will need to make some choices, and you will need some of the chutzpah that got me an afternoon snack with the first Prime Minister of Israel.

Good eating isn't something that is detached from everything else we do each day. It's part of a complete lifestyle influenced by the kitchen in which you cook, the attitude with which you cook, and the food you prepare. Developing a holistic, balanced, and healthy relationship with food must involve dealing with the emotions of change, and the fears, the impatience, and even the self-sabotage that can make the difference between success and failure.

It is also important to note that food and nourishment are not always one and the same. There are many foods that nourish us very little. Unfortunately, many of us are not always as sharp about distinguishing between these two as we need to be, especially when our cravings hit. If we're hankering after potato chips, we don't typically want to consider that

---

Well-chosen food, prepared with passion in the right environment, makes the body dance and the cells sing.

---

there may be little or no nutritional value until we're elbow deep into the bag—and by then it's too late.

I don't believe in deprivation, though. For me, food is to be enjoyed. Well-chosen food, prepared with passion in the right environment, makes the body dance and the cells sing. It's part of the joy of being alive. I encourage people to be disciplined but not neurotic about their eating. Having found a lot of truth in the old saying that "what you resist will persist," I advise clients that if they still love macaroni and cheese, then an occasional serving as a treat isn't going to be the end of the world.

My advice: don't just treat your cravings as the enemy and fight them. Instead, work with them. The way I explain it is that although cravings can be terribly damaging if they are given free reign, there is something honest and healthy at the heart of every one.

If you're craving sweets, you want some more sweetness in your life. If you're craving carbs, perhaps it's a feeling of fullness you're after. If you're craving alcohol, maybe it's the feeling of freedom and lightheartedness that a drink can give you.

We are not wrong to desire a sense of sweetness, a feeling of fullness, or a level of lightheartedness. The trouble is that many people just respond at a surface level and never delve deep enough to find out what they're really looking for. As a result, they settle for stuffing themselves with junk instead of getting the real nourishment their body is calling for.

So just remember, moderation!

A New Approach

What you choose to eat will, literally, be a matter of personal taste. That's why I don't recommend one diet plan for everyone. I advise people to cook and eat what their body tells them it needs. We all need to listen to what our bodies are saying. We each have a unique metabolism and digestive system. For example, after you eat pasta do you feel energetic or do you feel bloated and sluggish? Maybe pasta doesn't agree with you. For some of us wheat, which contains gluten, or dairy can be problematic. Try to eat meals and snacks that make you leave the table feeling full, nourished, and energized.

One thing I do encourage for everyone is an emphasis on fresh. Generally, eating "clean" food that is free of preservatives, hormones, or other additives is a healthier choice. The organic and "farm to table" movements are based on this principle. I love to use locally sourced items whenever possible.

Having traveled widely, I have picked up ideas and insights that have enabled me to develop expertise in a range of cuisines and cooking techniques, specializing in Mediterranean, kosher, paleo, vegetarian/vegan, and gluten-free dishes created by integrating traditional and new-wave cooking techniques.

Talk about how you want to be, not what you don't like about yourself.

Part of the reason for my success with clients, I believe, lies in the fact that I don't just encourage a new lifestyle, I encourage new language. I tell people to frame their hopes and goals positively, rather than speaking negatively about themselves. Talk about how you want to be, not what you don't like about yourself. That's just polluting the atmosphere with negative energy.

Most importantly, I never refer to "losing weight." Think about it: who wants to lose something? Usually that is a negative experience, isn't it? And if you lose something, you probably want to get it back. That's not a helpful "background track" to have running inside your head. Instead, I tell my clients to talk about releasing weight or letting go of weight—both of which have a much more positive vibe, suggesting a sense of freedom.

Before starting any kind of new eating program, take a day to indulge your cravings. I don't mean pig out, but if you're crazy for ice cream, have a couple of scoops. If you're lusting for pizza, enjoy a slice or two. Now is the time to do it. You're about to start out on a new journey and I don't want you to do it with any sense of resentment or deprivation.

I am not a nutritionist nor a dietitian, though I have read widely about both areas and work with my clients' nutritionists and dietitians to create the best individual program. But I have learned it is critical to be aware of your body's unique metabolism.

Imagine sitting in front of a fireplace, enjoying the steady flame. Put too much wood on that fire all at once and it will be smothered. Put too little and it will go out. To keep it steady, you need to feed it steadily. It's the same with your body and your metabolism.

Don't let your "food flames" get too high or too low. Neither stuffing yourself nor starving yourself is pleasant, nor is it very healthy. Instead, keep your metabolism burning at a strong, steady rate. You may find this means eating smaller portions more regularly, rather than sitting down to a fuller plate less frequently.

I always make sure to give clients plenty of encouragement as they embrace a new food lifestyle. I remind them that our bodies have an incredible ability to adapt to new conditions. "You got used to eating poorly," I'll say, "so why not give yourself the opportunity to get used to eating really well?"

Often I will tell them a story that can be a humorous motivator. It's about a Jewish villager who went to see his rabbi to complain.

"Rabbi, my parents are moving in with my wife and kids," the man said. "We're so squeezed as it is. I just don't know what to do."

The rabbi asked if they had any livestock.

"Yes, a goat and a donkey," the farmer replied.

"Move them into the house too," the rabbi advised.

The man was confused. "I just told you we've got no space in the house," he said, "and you want me to bring in the goat and the donkey?"

"Trust me," the rabbi said. "Do as I say and see me after thirty days."

A month later the farmer returned, very upset. "It's awful in my house, Rabbi," he grumbled. "I've got my parents in there and the animals and I can hardly breathe."

You got used to eating poorly so why not give yourself the opportunity to get used to eating really well?

"Okay," the rabbi said, "now take the donkey and goat out."

The farmer did as he was told, and came back to the rabbi overjoyed.

"You can't believe how much space we have!" he proclaimed.

The moral: It's all about having the right perspective.

Better eating isn't just about weight. There are other great results. People get more energy.

Their skin stops breaking out and their hair is healthier—it doesn't split like it did. Because of the quality of the food they're eating, many people drink less coffee. Sometimes, they may not even realize they're doing it. They don't feel as tired and draggy as they used to, and so they forget about that next cup of coffee.

I get excited to see these different changes and how much joy they bring people. It's the most rewarding part of my work.

Eating with Intention

One caution: please don't treat this approach as a strict ideology, like the bible of eating. This is not a regimen you have to follow without any flexibility at all. It's something that needs to be comfortable enough for you to live with for the long term, as an ongoing way of life, not a temporary practice.

Get in touch with your body. If you start feeling bloated or have low energy, you know something's not right. Check on your portions. Are they too big or too small? Does your frequency of eating need to be adjusted? And take your time while you're eating. Remember you don't have to eat everything on your plate if you don't want it. Stop long

Listen to what your body is telling you.

enough to see if you are full. Listen to what your body is telling you.

Determine what your ideal weight is and then stick to it. What is your ideal weight? It is not something you will find on a chart somewhere. It's when you feel good about yourself, and how you look in the mirror. Without becoming paranoid, you can keep an eye on how things are going.

Try weighing yourself once a week. If you fluctuate up to three pounds, don't worry about it. That is totally natural. Remember, you could gain some muscle and weigh more as a result. Don't fixate on the number, get in touch and stay in touch with the feeling. And if you should "fall off the wagon," get up, brush yourself off, and climb back on again. We only fail when we stop trying.

Just as it is important to cook with intention, it is important to eat with intention. That means being present, being in the moment, paying attention to the surroundings, just as you do when preparing something in the kitchen.

Try to make sure you have time to focus on what you are eating. Apart from anything, this will avoid the danger of carelessly overeating. Now, savor the look, the aroma, the flavor. When possible, eat with your hands. That restores our intimate connection to food.

Also, be sure to enjoy those you get to share your meal with them. Eat happy, as Oz points out in *Relish*. "If we want to live well, today, tomorrow, and in the future," she writes, "we must pledge to eat happy so that our bodies are energized for the hard work ahead."

Put your smartphone away, switch off the TV, and talk with each other at meal time. Give both your food and those you are sharing it with your full attention.

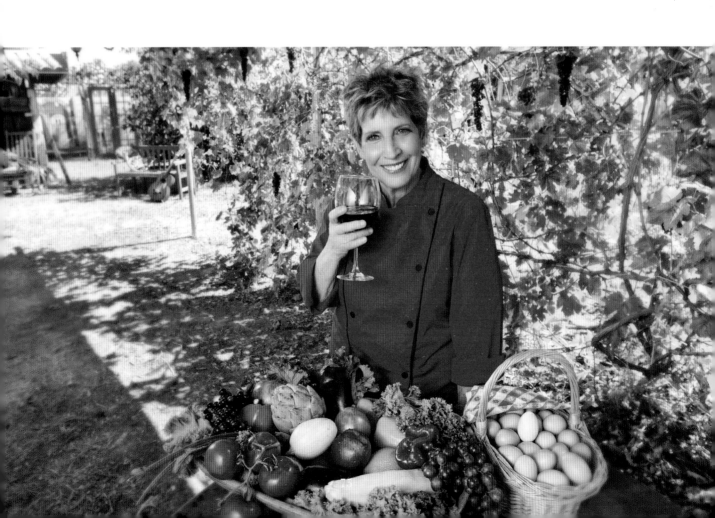

PIERCE BROSNAN'S MOROCCAN CHICKEN

Knowing their love for healthy eating, I was glad to be able to introduce Pierce Brosnan and his wife, Keely Shaye Smith, to a favorite Mediterranean-flavored dish of mine that combines nutritious and hearty eating.

(Serves 4)

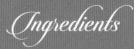

Ingredients

1 Tablespoon Extra Virgin Olive Oil

1 Medium Spanish Onion (diced)

1 14.5-oz. Can Fire-Roasted Tomatoes

6 Range-Free or Organic Skinless Chicken Thighs (with bone)

6-8 Fingerling Potatoes (cut in half)

½ Teaspoon Cayenne Pepper

1/8 Teaspoon Ground Cloves

½ Teaspoon Salt

½ Teaspoon Black Pepper

½ Cup Water

Spices, 1 teaspoon each of:

- Cumin
- Turmeric
- Coriander
- Cinnamon
- Curry Powder
- Garlic Powder
- Onion Powder

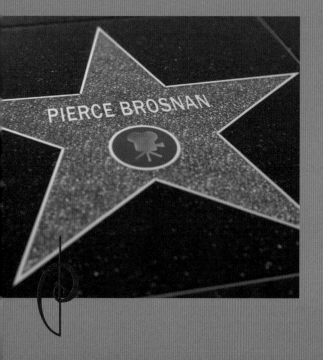

Instructions

1. In a heavy pot, heat up olive oil on medium and sauté onions until golden brown (approximately 5-8 minutes).

2. Add can of tomatoes, all the spices, and mix well. Cover pot and heat for additional 3-5 minutes on low simmer.

3. Remove lid and add the chicken, potatoes, and ½ cup water. Bring to low simmer, cover the pot, and cook for 35-45 minutes until chicken and potatoes are tender.

4. For serving, scoop onto each plate.

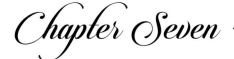

Chapter Seven

Developing and Maintaining a Healthy Food Lifestyle

PREPARING SOMEONE THEIR favorite food and seeing them enjoy it is rewarding, but it can be even more satisfying to serve them a surprise that they relish—maybe because the stakes are higher.

When you're making something with which they are familiar, you know what you are being judged against. When it's new there is a greater element of risk. Do you know them well enough to be able to "read" their likes and appetites?

One of the biggest dinner gambles I ever made was with a stake of more than $10,000. That is how much it cost to prepare an intimate eight-course meal for a famous actress-singer. As part of my work with her, I'd deliver healthy brown-bag lunches to the studio where she was filming a television series.

She came to me one day and told me she was inviting a top producer and his girlfriend over for a dinner with her and her boyfriend. She wanted a part in a movie the studio guy was involved in and hoped a fine meal might help seal the deal.

"I'm going to get this movie job and you are going to help me," she told me. "I want you to go over and beyond what you may be thinking. Don't tell me the menu, just surprise me. I trust you."

Well, that was exciting and scary at the same time. The challenge got my creative juices flowing. I had a month to prepare, designing just the right progression of small portions, from appetizers to desserts, and pairing each dish with the perfect wine. I ordered the best ingredients from one of Beverly Hills' top specialty food stores, and hired a sommelier to ensure the wines were exactly right.

Come the night, I joined the tuxedo-clad servers to introduce each course. "I'm Zipora," I said, "and I came all the way from Israel to prepare this meal for you." That got a laugh, and at the end of the meal I was brought back for a round of applause.

And my client got the part. *Phew!*

Sometimes it wasn't only my clients who were not sure what they were going to be eating for dinner. There were times when I did not know, either.

It was one thing to be able to cater well for The Kelly Family band members when we were at their home base in Cove, Ireland, a tiny, one-pub village about twenty minutes from Cork in the south of the country. Their favorites included Cornish hen and eggs Benedict. It was another matter when we were out on the road.

At that time, cities like Prague and Budapest that were just out from under Communist rule didn't always have the fresh vegetables I was familiar with. I had to use local produce I didn't know well, and still make it taste delicious and nourishing.

How did I do it? Intuition mostly, and sticking with the core principles of eating healthy. If you can't find romaine lettuce, it's not such a leap to replace it with some other green leafy vegetable that is available. In Croatia, for example, the street markets didn't carry asparagus, green beans, spinach, or zucchini—all vegetables that were an established part of the band's diet. But because Croatia is on the Adriatic coast, several kinds of seaweed vegetables were available.

From town to town and market to market, I didn't know what would be available. Sometimes even after I cooked the meal, I still didn't know the name of some of the items I had used in the meal. Band members would tell me a particular dish was delicious and ask me what was in it. All I could answer was, "Don't ask," with a smile.

Those rock tour travel experiences emphasized the importance of flexibility, and have helped me guide many other clients through the challenge of sticking with a program that sustains a healthy body weight and nutrition in the face of the challenges and uncertainties life often throws our way—whether we are at home or on the road.

Firmness and Flexibility

Most people who travel aren't fortunate enough to have a private chef to take care of them. They have to rely largely on restaurants. But it is possible to stay consistent with your eating when away from home. It just takes a little more intention and effort.

Planning ahead is key—taking time to prepare ahead of departure will reduce the challenges you face. For instance, consider booking a room that has a small kitchen so you can prepare your own food. Build a little time into your schedule so you can visit a store and stock up on the things you will need.

If you have to eat out, you don't need a restaurant with a low-carb or low-fat menu, ideal though that may be. But you do have to be specific about what food you want and how you want it prepared. It shouldn't be difficult to find a restaurant that can grill a piece of beef, chicken, or fish for you. Ask the server to have the chef prepare the meat or fish how you'd normally eat it at home.

If you're going for beef, choose filet mignon—it's the leanest cut. Always ask the server to request that the chef grill the meat, so there is no need for butter. Just to be absolutely sure, request No butter. You'll also want to be clear about No sauce. Don't worry about blandness. There's plenty the cook can do with spices alone to make your meat or fish delicious.

Add to this a steamed green vegetable and a small salad with a low-calorie dressing on the side. If there's no low-cal dressing, go for balsamic vinegar and olive oil. Now you've got a great meal without sacrificing your eating goals. You can even have dessert. Ask for a serving of fresh fruit like strawberries, melon, or peaches to top off your meal.

If you aren't taking care of yourself adequately, you're not going to be able to function at your best for very long.

We travel for different reasons and each kind of trip has its own mindset. What's important is that you don't put it ahead of your health and well-being. Take business travel as an example: you can be so focused on the work you need to get done that you neglect yourself and your own needs. But that's a short-sighted view. If you aren't taking care of yourself adequately, you're not going to be able to function at your best for very long.

Remember, your body is like a fireplace. You want to feed it fuel at a steady rate. Keeping with your aim of eating something every two to three hours may mean carrying some easy snacks with you. An apple, cheese sticks, or sliced veggies in a little travel cooler to keep everything fresh can provide what you need.

If you are taking a trip for pleasure, the temptation can be to take a vacation from healthy eating as well. Indulging yourself a little or trying something new is okay, but don't go overboard.

When traveling for business or fun, the biggest obstacle to good eating typically is time—either not enough for you to cater well for yourself, or too much so that you eat more than you should. On family visits, the biggest obstacle can sometimes be people!

I'm not suggesting that your family doesn't want you to be healthy. In most families, eating is a ritual, an almost sacred event. The way your family eats today is probably the way you used to eat back then, when you were with them—the old way. But now you have adopted a different approach. Here is where planning ahead can help: let them know beforehand how you have changed the way you eat, and ask for their help.

Usually they will be willing to accommodate you. Be aware, though, that becoming healthier and happier is your goal and others around you may not understand how important it is for you to eat healthy. They may even seem hurt or upset that you aren't indulging in the food the way you used to when you would visit.

For whatever reason, there may be occasions when it's almost impossible to escape everything you shouldn't eat. In these situations, my advice is: don't be extreme. Don't say no to everything, but don't overdo it either. You can accommodate someone's feelings without completely surrendering. Just say thank you and have a taste.

Creating a Team

For some people, the big obstacle they face in making a lasting change is internal. Deep down, they think they don't deserve the new life they are close to reaching, that somehow they are unworthy. And they quietly punish themselves. Others are scared they won't be able to maintain their new level, so they avoid the issue by making sure they never get there in the first place.

One client, a multi-millionaire businessman, dropped his weight by thirty-five pounds in less than four months through his new eating program. But then, in sight of his fifty-pound weight reduction goal, he began faltering. He would tell me he wanted to skip one week, then another. He claimed it was because he was traveling on business.

Finally, during a coaching session, I asked him about it. He admitted that it wasn't the travel—he was just more comfortable with what he knew, being overweight, than what lay ahead.

I challenged him, pointing out that he had not been afraid to go into the unknown in building a series of successful businesses; why not apply the same determination in regards to his health? If he wavered now, I warned, chances are he would in time slip all the way back to where he had been.

In the end, what helped this client press on through was encouraging him to pursue his goal not just for himself but also for his daughter, with whom I was also working.

Now thirteen, she had been overweight most of her life, and this was becoming more of an issue for her as she entered her teen years. Recognizing that if he slipped up he would be setting a poor example for his daughter, my client found the motivation to keep going after all.

This is why it can be helpful to have a team approach. You need people who are on your side, sharing and supporting your goals. As the song says, they can be the wind beneath your wings on those days when you are tired of flapping.

You might want to work with a lifestyle coach to keep you sharp. Or maybe consider spending some time with a therapist to look at certain bad habits or thought patterns that may have been in place since childhood. Don't be discouraged if you need some help in staying on track. We all need to be encouraged to make lifestyle changes permanent. Creating a support team around you is a great way to make sure you can get the right advice when you need it.

A little accountability can help too. I have a client who used to send me postcards when she traveled, letting me know how good she was doing on her eating. That was her motivation. She knew I cared and was proud to hear of her success and support her struggles.

Always keep in mind the long view. Remember that real transformation isn't temporary; it's forever. Like any lifestyle change, if it's worth starting, it's worth continuing. When you experience the real joy of eating, you'll want to feel that way all the time.

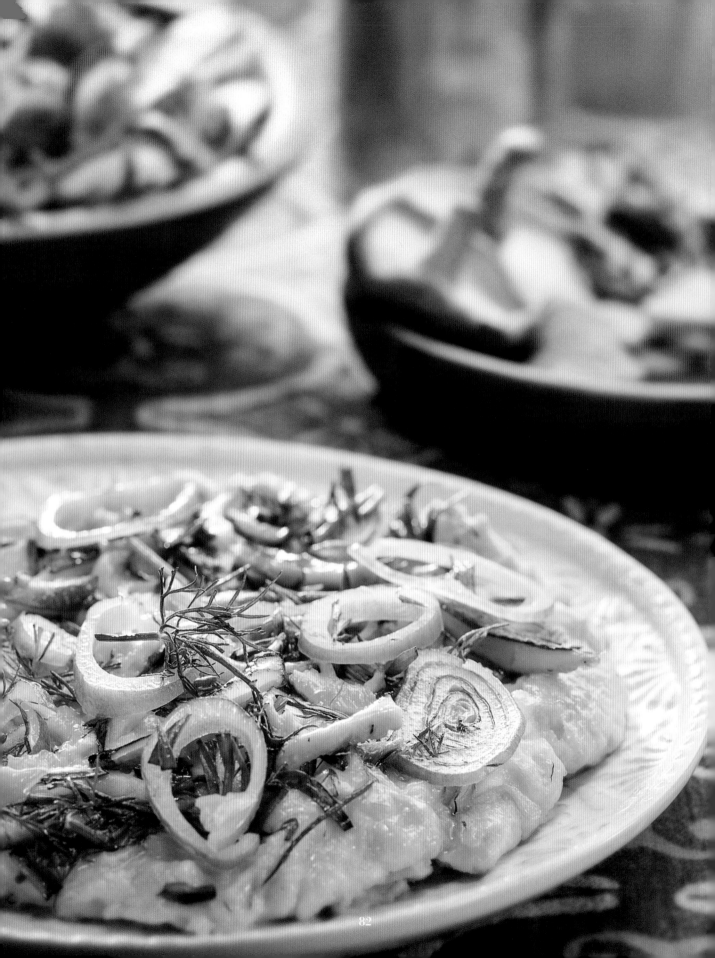

MARIAH CAREY'S LATE-NIGHT FRITTATA

When Mariah called me after one of her concerts on the *Rainbow* tour, unable to sleep and asking for something to eat, I knew that it needed to be something that would be satisfying, soothing, and also that would sit lightly on her stomach.

(Serves 2)

Ingredients

2 Teaspoons Virgin Olive Oil

2 Tablespoons Butter

4 Large Eggs

1/4 Teaspoon Dry Thyme

Salt and Black Pepper to taste

1 Cup Wild Mushrooms (thickly sliced)

1/2 Shallot (thinly sliced)

2 Tablespoons Half & Half Cream (or Almond Milk)

1 Tablespoon Chopped Parsley

Instructions

1. In 8-inch non-stick skillet, heat up 1 teaspoon of olive oil and 1 teaspoon of butter on medium heat.

2. Add the wild mushrooms, thyme, salt and pepper to taste. Sauté for 5-8 minutes until the liquid evaporates. Add mushrooms to a bowl and set aside. Wipe the skillet with paper towel for use again.

3. Whisk the eggs, salt and pepper. Slowly add the half & half cream (or almond milk.)

4. Using the skillet again, heat up 1 tablespoon butter on medium heat.

5. Add egg mixture; cook for approximately 2 minutes.

6. Spread mushrooms on top of the frittata and then add shallots. Salt and pepper to taste.

7. Cook for 6-8 minutes until almost set.

8. Take off heat, cover and let sit for another 2-3 minutes until set.

9. Decorate with parsley.

10. Cut in wedges and serve.

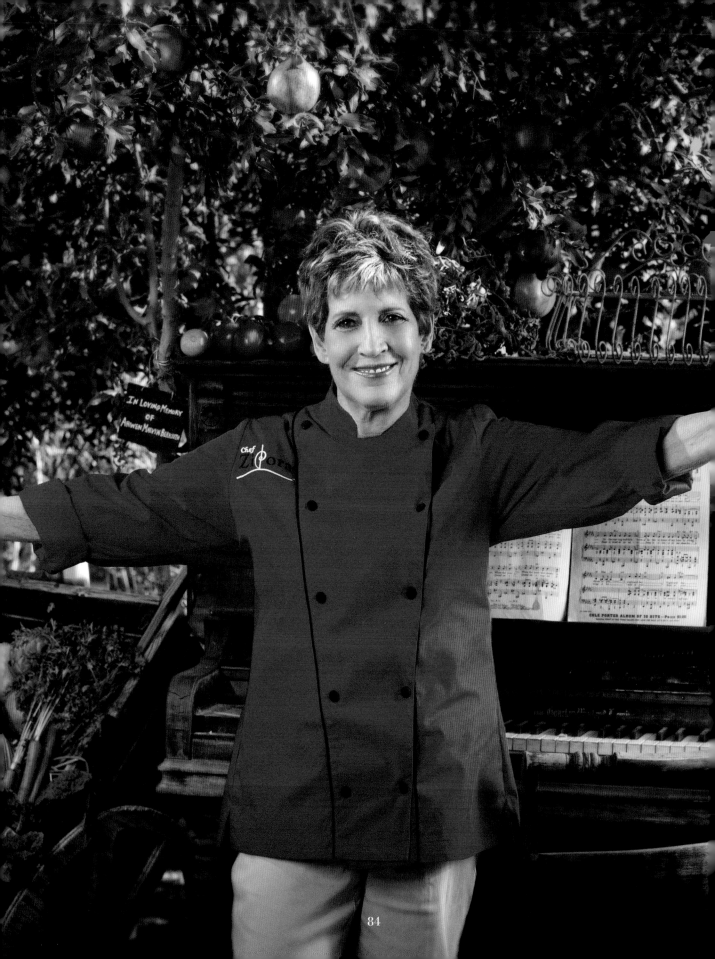

84

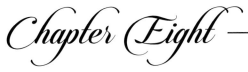

Chapter Eight

Music, the Secret Sauce

THERE IS A DEEP connection between food and music. I think writer Gregory David Roberts describes it well this way: "Food is music to the body, music is food to the heart." When we put the two together well, something magical happens.

Experimental psychologist Charles Spence, at Oxford University in England, has coined the word "gastrophysics" to describe the study of how all our senses—smell, texture, and sound, as well as taste—affect how we experience the food we eat.

"The atmosphere, the sights, the sounds, the smell, even the feel of the chair we happen to be sitting on (not to mention the size and shape of the table itself) all influence our perception and/or our behavior, however subtly," he writes in *Gastrophysics: The New Science of Eating.*

He notes how high-pitched music has been found to enhance the fruit notes people detect in wine. Often "the more we like the music, the more we enjoy the taste of the food or drink consumed while listening to that music," he says. And when people dine while listening to fast music, they tend to eat more quickly, as they do when the music is loud—in part because they don't talk as much. When the music is slower, they drink more.

"Mindful (or attentive) eating and drinking is important," Spence says, "and anything that we can do to make ourselves more aware of what we are consuming is going to help in terms of increased enjoyment, enhanced delivery of multi-sensory stimulation, and quite possibly increased satiety too."

Spence's research partner, experimental chef Jozef Youssef, has taken some of what they have learned so far and created The Gastrophysics Experience, a restaurant in London where guests can enjoy a multi-sensory dining experience. His thirteen-course meal is augmented by sights, sounds, and smells—the table cloth changes color during the evening—intended to enrich the flavor and enjoyment of offerings such as "Flavors of the Earth" (mushroom, cassava, and pumpernickel), and "An Education in Umami" (Parmesan, mushroom, and licorice).

85

I was fascinated to learn about Chef Youssef's experiment because it in many ways mirrors a unique multi-sensory experience I have developed in Phoenix, focused around food and music. I call this new experience my Ultimate Party. This is a one-of-a-kind dining event that offers guests the best from start to finish—where I prepare the best food in the best environment, accompanied by the best wine pairings along with live, classically inspired piano entertainment; all enjoyed in the best surroundings.

Catering for small groups in private homes or special locations in the Phoenix area and throughout the United States, I partner with two friends to ensure the perfect selections and settings. International Sommelier Lizbeth Congiusti, known as "The Sassy Sommelier" for her lively manner and storytelling abilities, brings her wine expertise to choosing just the right variety of grapes to serve with each course. Hungarian-born concert pianist and internationally renowned composer Peter Vamos, a former restaurateur, adds the finishing touch, playing improvisations and his own work with flourish as guests eat. One of these events, for a small group at the home of the head of a Phoenix-area television studio, was broadcast locally.

Fun as these events are, I'd love for more people to experience the same heightened enjoyment of combining music and food. That's why I commissioned and helped produce a music CD for people to listen to as they prepare food, carefully selected and played to help the chef find their "sweet spot."

Because it bypasses our intellect, music has a unique ability to touch us in our deepest emotions.

You could say that music is the secret sauce of good food—from its production to its preparation and consumption. You may have read how some farmers play music to their livestock to boost their milk yield and to improve the quality of the meat, as well using it to stimulate crop growth.

We are learning more about how music affects humans too. Studies have shown how it can lower stress and anxiety, improve memory, decrease pain levels, and increase attention—

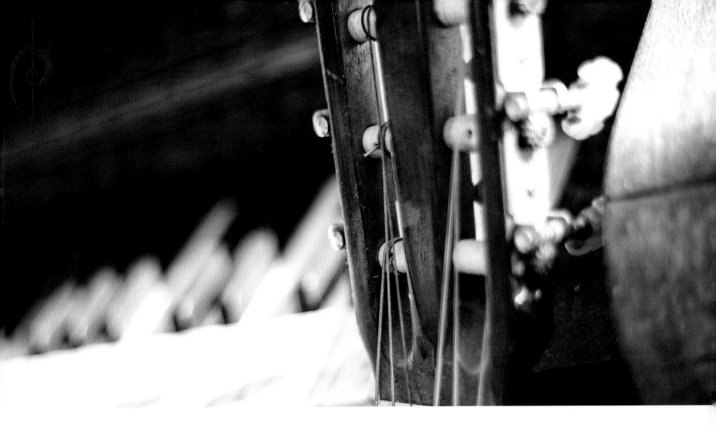

not to mention provide inspiration and motivation.

Classical music is particularly beneficial, it appears. One experiment found that people who listened to classical music had lower blood pressure than those who didn't. And some researchers believe classical music heightens our brains' ability to problem-solve.

Because it bypasses our intellect, music has a unique ability to touch us in our deepest emotions. It goes beyond the mind, straight to our heart. Beethoven put it this way: "Music is a higher revelation than all wisdom and philosophy. Music is the electrical soil in which the spirit lives, thinks and invents."

In *The Mozart Effect for Children: Awakening Your Child's Mind, Health, and Creativity, with Music*, Don Campbell, a musician and educator, looks into the benefits of music for education and health. He tells of research that shows how music relieves stress, encourages social interaction, stimulates language development, and improves motor skills among young children.

In addition, he says that music stimulates verbal skills and helps with study habits. There is also evidence that in the same way it communicates emotions, music helps create bonds that can alleviate symptoms of autism.

"It is amazing to think that music and rhythmic verbal sounds, which have been available to us throughout our lives, can have such a powerful effect on the mind and body," Campbell writes.

'Innergizing' Your Cooking

All kinds of music can touch us in some way, but classical music in particular seems to have the ability to reach deeply inside. It has been found, for example, that listening to classical music enhances the activity of genes involved in the secretion of dopamine, the "feel good" chemical released in our body, and serotonin, which regulates our moods. An article at Primephonic.com described it this way, "Simply put, our brains are programmed to be happier when we listen to music."

The brilliant physicist Albert Einstein liked to play classical music, especially pieces by Mozart, as he worked on his theories. It is said that Thomas Jefferson, the main author of the Declaration of Independence, would break from his work on the document to play the violin because it helped him think. Many other famous people in history have told of how classical music has enriched their lives in some way.

I asked Neil Argo to help me bring that same kind of inspiration to the kitchen. He has created a beautiful suite of piano music, weaving in elements of Bach, Handel, Vivaldi, and Beethoven to elevate the listener as they prepare food.

Another CD I have produced for children features classical music by Mozart over which are spoken simple affirmations to further inspire young listeners, like "I love myself," "I love good food," and "I love to help cook." I believe these simple words will further enrich the lives of younger people by helping them have more awareness of and a more positive attitude towards food. After all, words are very powerful. In the book of Genesis it says "God said, 'Let there be light,' and there was light": that's powerful!

If classical music is the most singular impactful style, then within it baroque appears to have its own special dimension. Some people say baroque music is especially good at stimulating deep focus and concentration because of the way it generally pulses at between fifty and eighty beats per minute, enhancing our alpha brainwave state.

I remember reading about an experiment in which some researchers placed a plant next to a speaker through which they played baroque music for a month. Over time, the plant wound itself round the speaker, as if in a hug. Then they switched the selection to heavy metal music, and in due course the plant turned away, almost as if it were trying to cover its ears.

However, in many busy restaurant kitchens, where there's a lot of pressure, they play rock music to keep everyone pumped up and on their toes. It does provide a certain physical buzz, but I don't believe it releases the emotional or inner energy that we want to share through the food we prepare for others.

With that in mind, I knew I needed to find some sort of middle way for my music CD for chefs. So I commissioned composer Neil Argo, the award-winning creator of atmospheric music for the likes of television's *Beverly Hills 90210, Melrose Place*, (The New) *Mission Impossible* and *Wild America*, and movies such as *The Legends of Nethiah* and *Chasing the Green*, to blend the heart of baroque with a techno beat that I believe both energizes and "innergizes" the listener.

...pouring love and care into the meals we share with others,

we nourish them both physically and emotionally...

Working with Neil, I learned more about the amazing connection between music and food. With his own understanding of the strong food-music relationship, I believe that through our collaboration, *Music for a Delicious Life*, we have been able to produce some truly inspirational music for people to play. As they listen while they prepare food in a well-harmonized kitchen, I believe it will help them do so at optimal performance.

In this way, pouring love and care into the meals we share with others, we nourish them both physically and emotionally so they can live healthy and happy lives that enrich others too.

What an exciting thought, that we can be part of making the world a better place from our kitchens!

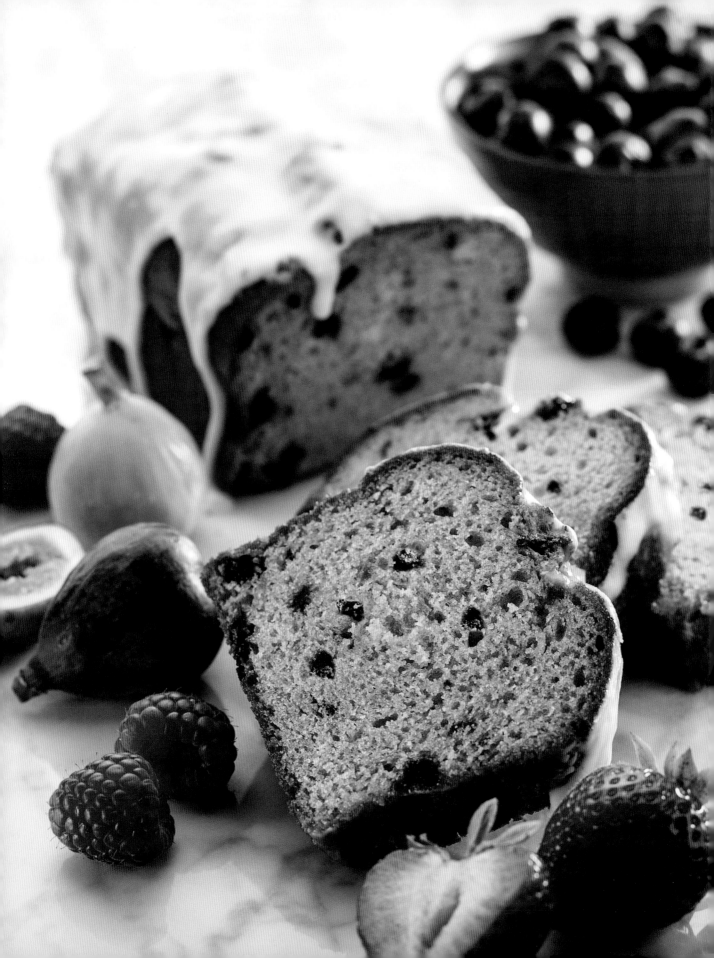

THE KELLY FAMILY'S BLUEBERRY LOAF

This was another favorite of The Kelly Family, usually requested over the weekend. I would joke and tell them it was only made to reward them for good behavior!

(Serves 10)

Ingredients

CAKE

1-1/2 Cups All-Purpose Flour

1/2 Teaspoon Salt

1 Teaspoon Baking Powder

1 Cup Sugar

2 Tablespoons Lemon Peel

3/4 Cup Buttermilk

1/2 Cup Coconut Oil

2 Large Eggs

1 Tablespoon Fresh Lemon Juice

1 Teaspoon Vanilla Extract

1 Cup Fresh Blueberries

LEMON GLAZE

1 Cup Powdered Sugar

2 Tablespoons Fresh Lemon Juice

Instructions

1. Preheat oven to 350° F.

2. Spray 8-½-inch x 4-inch bread pan with olive oil.

3. In a bowl, mix together the flour, salt, and baking powder

4. In another bowl, combine the sugar and lemon peel. Rub together with your fingers until the mixture feels like sand. Then add to the dry ingredients and mix well.

5. In another bowl, combine the buttermilk, coconut oil, eggs, lemon juice, and vanilla extract. Mix well and then slowly add to the dry ingredients.

6. Gently fold in the fresh blueberries. Don't over-mix!

7. Pour the mixture into the bread pan.

8. Bake 65-70 minutes until a toothpick comes out clean.

9. Cool on rack for 15 minutes then remove the cake from the loaf and continue to cool.

10. Make the lemon glaze: In a bowl, mix together the powdered sugar and lemon juice. Spread onto the cooled blueberry loaf.

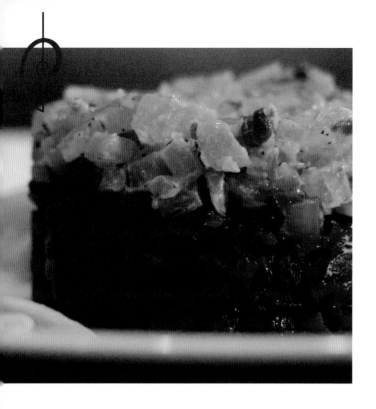
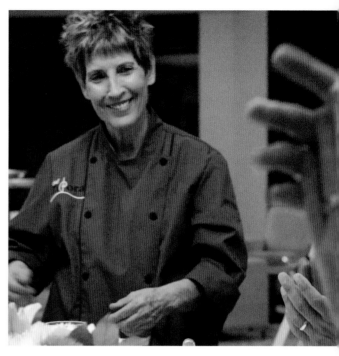
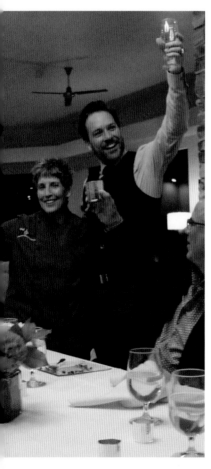
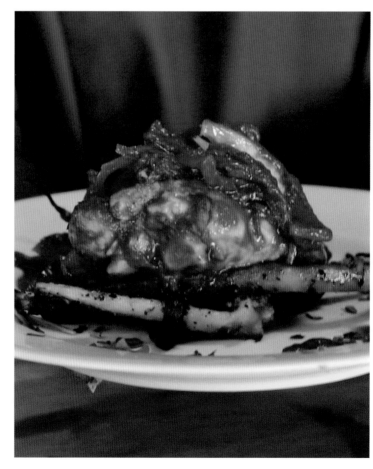
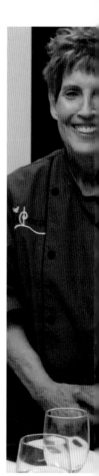

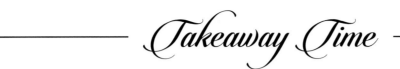

Takeaway Time

I HOPE THAT in reading this book you have been inspired to practice the sort of intentional food preparation and eating which nourishes the whole person—body, mind, and spirit. Now I want to leave you with something that will assist you in incorporating all you've read into your life.

Ideally, I'd welcome you to a special dinner where you could personally experience all I have talked about—food prepared and presented with love and care and enjoyed in a perfect environment under a banner of music.

Sadly that's not possible, but I have come up with the next best thing—your virtual seat at just such a meal. Follow the link here or at my website, www.chefzipora.com, and you can join me and some friends for a wonderful celebration. With the help of the latest interactive technology, you'll almost feel like you can reach out for some of the food you'll see me preparing and sharing with a small group in a beautiful home.

As well as seeing how I prepare the meal, you will be able to experience the way in which some of the special music by Neil Argo and Peter Vamos enhances the appreciation and enjoyment of eating. I'm so confident you will want to replicate what you experience that I am including the recipes at the end of this section so you can share the experience with family and friends.

I have more for you at my website too. You've read about how I teamed up with my talented friends to create the Ultimate Party, and you can find details about how we can throw one especially for you.

Also on my website you will find more menus and recipes for your everyday life. You can also hear some of the original music Neil Argo and Peter Vamos have composed and created, and obtain copies of the CDs we have produced to enhance your own food preparation and enjoyment.

Life is a constant journey of discovery, and I am excited to be able to let you know what else I learn in the days ahead. Don't forget to follow my blog on the website and stay in touch with me on my Facebook, Twitter and Instagram accounts. And finally, you can follow my musical journey on the Chef Zipora Enterprise YouTube channel, www.youtube.com/channel/UC21s6uHDw2PptyOEMdh0n_A

I would love to hear from you too. Please let me know what you have learned about intentional cooking and eating and what it has meant in your life. Tell me what you'd like to know more about.

May your food preparation be nourishing, your meals enriching, and your life harmonious!

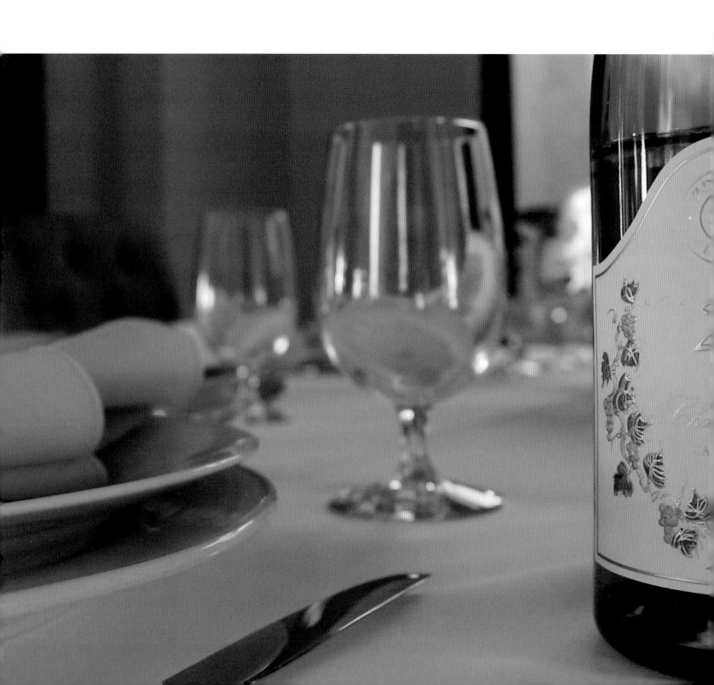

MY SPECIAL DINNER

FRESH APRICOT WITH GOAT CHEESE AND HONEY
(Serves 4)

Ingredients

8 Fresh Apricots (cut in half)

6 oz. Goat Cheese

1-1/2 Teaspoons Honey

1-1/2 Teaspoons Fresh Rosemary (chopped)

1 Teaspoon Fresh Thyme (chopped)

1/2 Cup Whole Roasted Almonds

Instructions

1. In a bowl, mix together the goat cheese, honey, rosemary, and thyme. Fill the center of each apricot with the mixture. Add the roasted almonds to the top of the filling.

2. Decorate with chervil herbs or chive and serve on a plate.

MOROCCAN ORANGE AND BLACK OLIVE SALAD
(Serves 4)

Ingredients

3 Tablespoons Good Quality Virgin Olive Oil

1-1/2 Tablespoons Fresh Lime Juice

1 Tablespoon Honey

1 Clove Garlic (smashed)

1/2 Teaspoon Cumin

1/4 Teaspoon Smoked Paprika

1/8 Teaspoon Red Pepper Flakes

1/2 Teaspoon Salt

6 Oranges

1 Cup Black Olives (sliced)

2 Tablespoons Chopped Parsley

Instructions

1. In a small bowl, mix together the olive oil, lime juice, honey, garlic, cumin, paprika, red pepper flakes, and salt.

2. Remove all peel from the oranges in a circular motion and slice each one horizontally.

3. Arrange the orange slices in one layer on the center of each of the 4 plates.

4. Spread the olives and drizzle oil on top.

5. Decorate with parsley and serve.

MY SPECIAL DINNER

ROASTED RED AND GOLDEN BEETS TARTARE

(Serves 4)

Ingredients

1 Red Beet (finely diced)

1 Golden Beet (finely diced)

3 Tablespoons Olive Oil

1/2 Cup Red Onion (minced)

6 Tablespoons Parsley

2 Tablespoons Capers

4 Tablespoons Dijon Mustard

2 Teaspoons Worcestershire Sauce

Salt and Black Pepper to taste

Instructions

1. Preheat oven to 400° F.

2. Cut the top off each beet. Wrap the red and golden beets in separate aluminum foil and add a splash of olive oil. Roast for 45-60 minutes, or until soft. Then let cool.

3. When the beets are cool enough to handle, peel off and separate the skin.

4. Place the finely diced red and golden beets in two separate bowls.

5. To each bowl, add ¼ cup onion, 3 tablespoons parsley and 1 tablespoon capers

6. In a small bowl, add the Dijon mustard and Worcestershire sauce, slowly adding the olive oil. Then divide the mixture in half and add to each bowl of red and golden beets. Salt and pepper to taste.

To serve, add the red beets and add yellow beets together in a circle on the middle of a plate. Decorate with parsley.

MY SPECIAL DINNER

THE ULTIMATE MOROCCAN CHICKEN

(Serves 6)

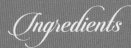

Ingredients

2 Teaspoons each of:

- Cinnamon
- Cumin
- Coriander

1 Teaspoon Salt

1 Teaspoon Black Pepper

1 Teaspoon Turmeric

1 Teaspoon Red Pepper Flakes

1/2 Teaspoon Clove Powder

1/2 Teaspoon Smoked Paprika

1 Red Onion (sliced)

3 Cloves Garlic (thinly sliced)

2 Tablespoons Olive Oil

2 Cups Tomato Juice

12 Dried Apricots

6 Chicken Thighs with bones (skinless)

Instructions

1. In a bowl, mix the spices together (cinnamon, cumin, coriander, black pepper, turmeric, red pepper flakes, clove power, paprika). Then rub some of the mixture onto the 6 pieces of chicken and set aside.

2. Heat a deep frying pan to almost smoking, turn up heat to medium and then add olive oil for 30 seconds. Then add chicken thighs.

3. Roast chicken thighs on both sides until they are golden brown, about 6-8 minutes. Add the red onion and cook for another 3 minutes. Then add garlic and cook for another 6 minutes, until onions are soft.

4. Add tomato juice and cook for another 1-2 minutes.

5. Add any remaining spice mixture. Cover fry pan and turn heat to low, then cook for another 30-35 minutes until chicken is tender. Add 12 dried apricots. Cook for 5-7 minutes

BAILEYS AFFOGATO DESSERT

(Serves 6)

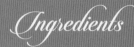
Ingredients

6 Shots Strong Hot Brewed Espresso

18 oz. (or 12 scoops) High Quality French Vanilla Ice Cream

1-1/2 Cups Baileys Irish Cream Liqueur

Instructions

1. Brew espresso.
2. In 6 large clear dessert glasses, add 2 scoops of ice cream.
3. Divide the Baileys evenly and pour onto the ice cream.
4. Fill each cup with the espresso and serve.

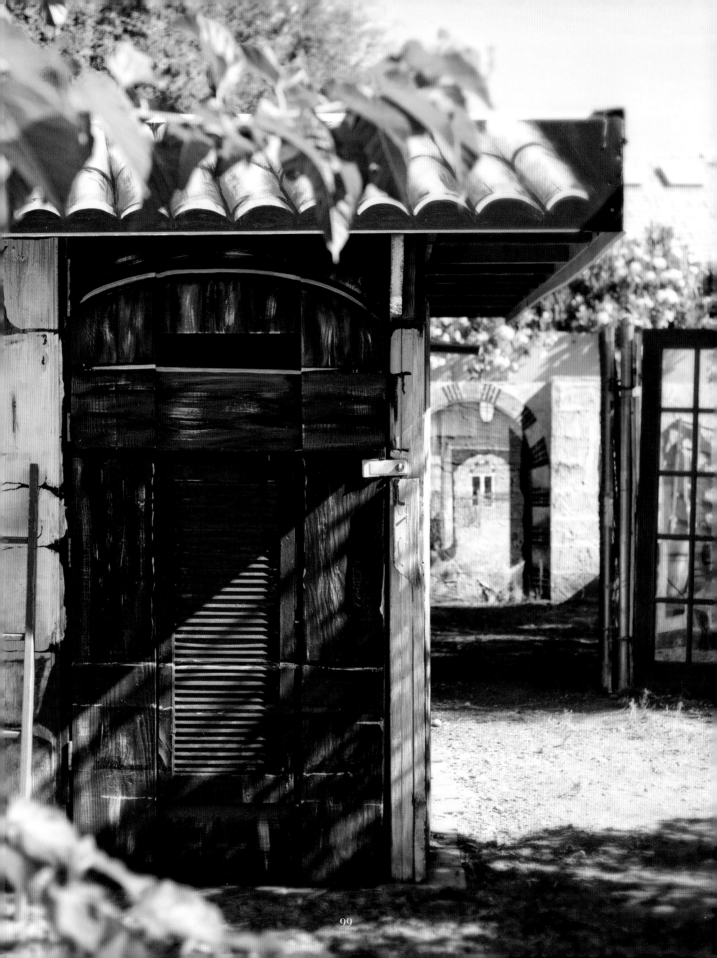

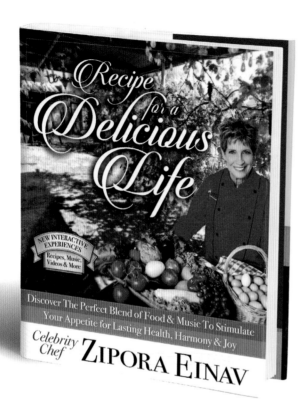

To order additional copies
of the book go to
www.chefzipora.com

If you're a fan of this book,

WILL YOU HELP ME SPREAD THE WORD?

It is my desire to see people all over the world experience the joy and pleasure of cooking, eating and living well. Will you help me?

Here are some practical things you can do…

- Post a 5-Star review on Amazon, Goodreads and other places that come to mind.

- Write about the book on your Facebook, Twitter, Instagram, Pinterest, Google+, any social media sites you regularly use.

- If you blog, consider referencing the book, or publishing an excerpt from the book with a link back to my website.

- Take a photo of yourself with your copy of the book. Post it on your social media – email me a copy as well!

- Recommend the book to friends – word of mouth is still the more effective form of advertising.

- When you're in a bookstore, ask them if they carry the book. The book is available through all major distributors, so any bookstore that does not have it in stock can easily order it.

- Do you know a journalist or media personality who might be willing to interview me or write an article based on the book? If you will email mail me your contact, I will gladly follow up.

- Purchase additional copies to give as gifts.

MAKE MAGIC HAPPEN IN YOUR HOME AND YOUR HEART

I have found that music is often the "secret ingredient" that makes preparing, serving and tasting food more enjoyable. I have partnered with my friend, famed movie and television score composer Neil Argo to bring you this CD of original classical music with a techno background.

Visit www.chefzipora.com/shop

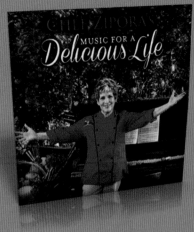

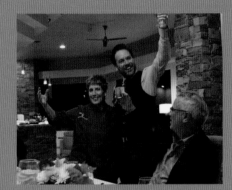

WHEN YOU WANT TO CREATE A TRULY MEMORABLE EVENT

CHEF ZIPORA'S ULTIMATE PARTY

Whether you are hosting the ultimate office party, engagement party, business meeting, fundraising banquet, if you want to raise the bar and truly make a statement, hire Zipora to cater that event.

Experience the magic created when gourmet food is combined with the finest wine selections and storytelling, topped off with distinctive improvisational piano entertainment.

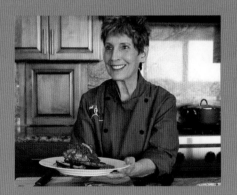

CALL ME WHEN YOU'RE HUNGRY

Do you have a busy household that could use a personal chef to prepare healthy, delicious meals each week or a special event – anniversary, birthday, family reunion, retirement or maybe a business meeting – that you are planning? Let's connect and talk about your needs – and I'll get started!

SPEAKING AND GUEST INTERVIEWS

If you are part of an organization that has guest speakers or you know of an organization who might want me to speak, lead a workshop or make a presentation, then please contact me at:

www.chefzipora.com

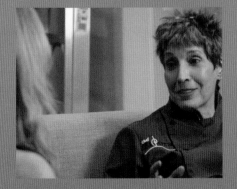

Chef Zipora
ENTERPRISE
™